The Lupus Journey

Shedding Light on the Challenges and Triumphs

Dr. Amanda Bates

Copyright

TABLE OF CONTENT

INTRODUCTION

Getting Around the Lupus Terrain

Millions of people worldwide are impacted by the complex disorder known as lupus, which lurks in the shadowy corners of medicine's vast tapestry. The ripple effects of lupus become apparent as we travel, affecting not just the individuals who bear its burden but also the entire fabric of their families and communities. This introduction provides an entry point into the world of lupus, where knowledge, understanding, and resilience come together.

Lupus's Effects on People and Families

Lupus is a force that alters life in unforeseen ways; it is more than just a medical diagnosis. The effects of lupus can range from a chronic joint ache to erratic flare-ups that interfere with everyday activities. The disease has a profound and deeply personal impact. This section explores the personal stories of people living with lupus, illuminating the obstacles they encounter and the resilience they muster to achieve wellness.

Lupus affects not just the individual but also families, creating a web of resilience and shared experiences. Experiencing a loved one's journey through the intricacies of an autoimmune disorder can be emotionally taxing, but it can also be characterized by empathy, understanding, and a shared will to meet the obstacles head-on. In this investigation, we examine the connections that bind lupus-affected families, highlighting the need of maintaining a unified front in the face of hardship.

Goals and Purpose of the Book

Why take on this investigation on lupus? The goal that drives the pages that follow is explained in this section. It is an appeal to action, asking readers to accompany us on our trek through the maze that is lupus. This book tries to be a compass in the huge world of information, whether you are a person with lupus, a caregiver, a healthcare professional, or someone just looking for information.

This book covers more ground than only the clinical aspects of lupus. Our journey recognizes the emotional, psychological, and social aspects of lupus that come together to form a whole story, even as we delve into the medical nuances of the condition. This all-inclusive manual aims to empower lupus sufferers, their families, and the communities they affect by building understanding and resiliency.

Comprehending Lupus: A Range of Intricacy

Understanding the subtleties of lupus is essential before figuring out the next steps. This section reveals lupus as a spectrum of autoimmune illnesses by removing some of the layers of intricacy. Every variation of the disease presents unique difficulties, ranging from cutaneous lupus and lupus nephritis to systemic lupus erythematosus (SLE). We examine the unique traits of different kinds to give readers a basis for comprehending the variety of lupus manifestations.

The Environmental and Genetic Dance

The genesis of lupus is shaped by a dance between genetics and the environment. This section examines the genetic predispositions that may increase a person's risk of developing lupus. At the same time, we identify the environmental elements that are critical in initiating the disease. Understanding this complex dance helps readers comprehend the causes of lupus, which opens the door to educated conversations about management and prevention.

Symptoms and Outward Signs of Illness

Like a language the body speaks, lupus symptoms can be complex and varied. This section provides a vocabulary that decodes the messages that lupus transmits, from the obvious symptoms like joint pain and skin rashes to the more subdued ones like weariness and organ inflammation. Understanding the various ways the illness presents itself can help patients and those who care for them deal with its difficulties by raising understanding of the complexities involved.

Medical Diagnostics and Perspectives

Lupus diagnosis is like trying to solve a jigsaw puzzle with moving pieces. This section delves into the diagnostic standards and testing techniques used by medical experts to solve the mystery of lupus. In order to provide prompt and exact care, we emphasize the value of a collaborative and interdisciplinary approach as we navigate the complexity of the sometimes difficult path to an accurate diagnosis.

Healthcare Providers Associated with Lupus Management

The management of lupus is a symphony performed by a varied group of medical specialists. Experts in rheumatology, dermatology, nephrology, and mental health all contribute their knowledge to develop a well-rounded strategy for managing lupus. It is critical for readers to comprehend the responsibilities of these experts, and this section offers a thoughtful synopsis that encourages cooperation and shared accountability in the pursuit of wellbeing.

Treatment Strategies

Lupus treatment involves a personalized, detailed plan for each patient rather than a generic medication. This section gives readers a thorough grasp of all the options, from pharmaceutical interventions to new medicines and clinical trial involvement. Understanding the complexities of lupus care empowers people to make educated decisions, taking an active role in their care and determining their own route to wellness.

Encouraging Through Information: A guiding principle

Since information is a powerful tool for guiding people, this book aims to empower lupus sufferers and those who support them. The intention is to empower readers as we delve into the nuances of the illness and not just to enlighten them. By providing people with information, we hope to develop champions who take an active role in their care, make wise decisions, and push for greater understanding and awareness of lupus.

This introduction essentially establishes the framework for a thorough investigation of lupus. It invites readers to embark with us on an adventure that goes beyond the professional confines of a medical handbook. Our guide through the terrain of lupus is provided not only by the medical complexities but also by the individual experiences, resiliency, and group spirit that characterize the lupus community.

Chapter One

Comprehending Lupus: A Thorough

Examination

One example of the complex interplay between the human immune system and its complexity is the multifaceted autoimmune disease known as lupus. In our quest to comprehend lupus, we will explore its various forms and presentations, decipher the interaction between hereditary and environmental factors, and solve the diagnostic riddle that frequently accompanies the disease's early stages. This chapter provides readers with a thorough overview, enabling them to better comprehend and navigate the terrain of lupus.

1. Lupus Erythematosus Systemic (SLE)

The most common and complex type of lupus is called systemic lupus erythematosus (SLE). Because of its systemic nature, it can impact different organs and tissues, resulting in a wide range of symptoms. Common symptoms include fatigue, rashes on the skin, joint pain, and internal organ inflammation. The recognizable butterfly rash that spreads across the face frequently becomes a visual representation of SLE.

Comprehending SLE is like trying to understand the intricacies of a dynamic orchestra. When the immune system interprets healthy cells as alien invaders, it mistakesnly triggers an autoimmune reaction that spreads throughout the entire body. Because of this systemic involvement, diagnosis and treatment must take a multifaceted approach.

2. Lupus Cutaneous

The primary site of cutaneous lupus is the skin, and it manifests itself in a variety of dermatological ways. Subacute cutaneous lupus erythematosus (SCLE) frequently presents with photosensitive rashes, whereas discoid lupus erythematosus (DLE) causes coin-shaped skin lesions. A dermatological viewpoint is necessary to comprehend the subtleties of cutaneous lupus, highlighting the significance of rheumatologists and dermatologists working together to provide comprehensive care.

3. lupus arthritis

The kidney-affecting type of lupus called lupus nephritis presents a different set of difficulties. The kidneys, which are essential for eliminating waste and preserving fluid equilibrium, end up being the target of the autoimmune attack. Examining the implications for managing the disease as a whole as well as its renal manifestations is essential to comprehending the complexities of lupus nephritis.

Understanding the various forms of lupus paves the way for a more complex comprehension of the difficulties that people may experience. Each variation adds to the overall composition of the disease and symbolizes a distinct movement in the lupus symphony. This knowledge becomes essential when designing interventions to target particular symptoms and improve the quality of life for lupus patients.

Environmental and Genetic Factors

1. Predispositions Generic

The first stanza of the lupus symphony is genetics, which is vital in determining one's susceptibility to the illness. An increased risk of developing lupus is linked to specific genetic markers, such as certain types of the human leukocyte antigen (HLA), which suggests a genetic component in familial tendencies. But the genetic terrain of lupus is complex, involving several genes with different degrees of involvement.

Recognizing that lupus is a polygenic illness rather than a straightforward Mendelian trait is necessary to comprehend the genetic foundations of the disease. Numerous genes influence the likelihood of developing lupus by interacting with environmental factors and contributing to the overall genetic susceptibility. While genetic predispositions by themselves do not ensure the development of lupus, they do provide a favorable environment in which environmental stimuli may initiate the autoimmune reaction.

2. Environmental Stressors

The second stanza of the poem is devoted to environmental factors related to lupus, which introduce outside variables that may affect how the illness develops. Several environmental triggers, including hormones, medications, infections, and exposure to specific chemicals, have been linked to the development of lupus. Each person experiences the complex dance between genetics and environment in a unique way, which adds to the variation seen in lupus symptoms.

Comprehending the environmental triggers entails realizing that they can function as initiators or intensifiers of the autoimmune reaction. For instance, infections have the ability to activate the immune system and possibly cause flare-ups of lupus. Drug-induced lupus has been linked to medications, including antiepileptic drugs and some blood pressure medications. The course of lupus can also be influenced by hormonal fluctuations, such as those that occur during pregnancy or menopause.

Understanding how genetic predispositions and environmental triggers interact helps people and medical professionals understand the variables that lead to the development of lupus. This information serves as the foundation for targeted interventions and preventive measures meant to reduce the chance of lupus flare-ups or onset by modifying environmental exposures.

3. Symptoms and Outward Signs of Illness

Known as the great imitator, lupus presents a wide range of symptoms that can be mistaken for other illnesses. Deciphering the complex symphony of lupus symptoms is crucial to a precise diagnosis and successful treatment. Understanding the subtle differences between each symptom and its corresponding note in the autoimmune composition empowers both patients and healthcare professionals.

4. Stiffness and Pain in the Joints

The lupus symphony is frequently accompanied by joint pain and stiffness, which frequently mimic the signs of arthritis. The autoimmune response targets the synovium, the lining of the joints, causing inflammation, pain, and stiffness. Differentiating lupus-related joint symptoms from other types of arthritis and designing appropriate interventions require an understanding of their unique characteristics.

5. Manifestations on the Skin

Lupus is known for its involvement of the skin, and the disease's visual landscape is influenced by a variety of dermatological manifestations. SLE is characterized by the butterfly rash, a malar rash that spreads across the face. Rashes can result from photosensitivity reactions, in which the skin becomes extremely sensitive to sunlight. Coin-shaped lesions are a common presentation of discoid lupus erythematosus, highlighting the variety of skin manifestations associated with lupus.

6. Weary

The experience of having lupus is infused with fatigue, which clouds day-to-day activities. This ubiquitous feeling of exhaustion goes beyond everyday fatigue and frequently becomes the main theme of the lupus symphony. Investigating the links between lupus-related fatigue, anemia, and the psychological costs associated with managing a chronic illness is necessary to comprehend the complex nature of this fatigue.

7. Organ Participation

Lupus can affect almost every organ in the body; it is not just limited to the skin and joints. Lupus nephritis, or inflammation of the kidneys, can cause proteinuria and worsen kidney function. The symptoms of cardiac involvement can include myocarditis or pericarditis. The systemic nature of lupus is further highlighted by neurological symptoms, hematological abnormalities, and pulmonary complications.

Understanding the various forms of lupus is like trying to figure out a complicated musical score. Every note adds to the whole, and the combination of symptoms creates the distinct sound of every person's lupus experience. This knowledge is essential for healthcare professionals to diagnose patients because it helps them make the connections between symptoms and create specialized treatment plans.

Solving the Diagnostic Mysterium

1. Criteria for Diagnosis

Lupus diagnosis is like putting together a puzzle, each piece requiring careful thought. Certain clinical and immunological features must be present in order to meet the diagnostic criteria set forth by the American College of Rheumatology (ACR). These criteria, which call for a specific set of symptoms to be present in order to diagnose lupus, include immunological, musculoskeletal, mucocutaneous, and renal components.

Comprehending the diagnostic criteria necessitates acknowledging that lupus is not a universally applicable ailment. Although the criteria offer a structure, people with lupus can present with a wide range of symptoms due to its complexity. Rheumatologists, who are frequently the main gatekeepers in the diagnosis of lupus, manage this complexity by carrying out in-depth evaluations and taking into account each patient's distinct clinical presentation.

2. Antibodies against nuclei (ANAs)

An important piece of the lupus diagnostic puzzle is the role of antinuclear antibodies (ANAs). A sizable portion of lupus patients have these antibodies, which attack the body's own cell nuclei. ANAs, however, are not unique to lupus; they are also present in other autoimmune diseases. When ANAs are detected, additional research is prompted, directing medical professionals to look into more clinical and laboratory factors in order to make a conclusive diagnosis.

3. Multidisciplinary Method

Solving the diagnostic conundrum requires a multidisciplinary strategy. Specialists such as rheumatologists, dermatologists, nephrologists, and others work together to acquire information about the various ways that lupus manifests itself. Blood tests, imaging studies, and sometimes biopsies add more pieces to the diagnostic puzzle. Effective collaboration among healthcare providers is crucial for guaranteeing a thorough assessment and precise diagnosis.

A key component of this section is educating people about the diagnostic procedure. Through comprehension of the associated criteria and examinations, people take an active role in their diagnostic process. It becomes imperative to advocate for comprehensive evaluations and efficient communication with medical professionals in order to successfully navigate the diagnostic complexities associated with lupus.

Healthcare Providers Associated with Lupus Management

1. rheumatologists

The main designers of lupus care are rheumatologists, who specialize in musculoskeletal and autoimmune diseases. Their responsibilities go beyond diagnosis to include continuing supervision, modifying a course of treatment, and coordinating care with other professionals. For people with lupus, knowing the critical role rheumatologists play is essential, as these medical professionals take on a central role in their healthcare journey.

2. Dermatologists

Dermatologists are specialists in skin disorders, and cutaneous lupus patients benefit greatly from their involvement. A comprehensive approach to the management of lupus is ensured by acknowledging the distinct dermatological manifestations and working in conjunction with dermatologists. Working together, rheumatologists and dermatologists can effectively address the disease's systemic as well as skin-related aspects.

3. nephrologists

One kidney-related manifestation of lupus that brings nephrologists into the collaborative realm of lupus care is lupus nephritis. These experts concentrate on kidney function and are vital in the treatment of renal complications associated with lupus. The cooperation of nephrologists and rheumatologists is essential to providing patients with lupus nephritis with comprehensive care.

4. Experts in Mental Health

It is impossible to overstate the emotional toll that having a chronic illness like lupus takes. Therapists and psychologists are examples of mental health professionals who support lupus patients holistically. Taking care of psychological issues like stress, anxiety, and depression becomes crucial to managing lupus. Acknowledging the function of mental health specialists highlights the comprehensive aspect of lupus treatment.

5. Multidisciplinary Cooperation

A range of healthcare professionals are involved in the multidisciplinary nature of lupus care. By combining their knowledge, nurses, PTs, dietitians, and other experts create a comprehensive strategy for managing the various aspects of the illness. The collaborative efforts among these specialists guarantee that patients with lupus receive comprehensive and all-encompassing care.

In the context of lupus care, having a clear understanding of the roles played by different healthcare professionals promotes cooperation and shared accountability. People grow into capable advocates who actively interact with their medical team and understand the value of a coordinated strategy to manage the intricacies of lupus.

Methods of Therapy: A Guide to Well-Being

1. Pharmaceutical Interventions

The mainstay of lupus care is pharmacological interventions, which are designed to manage symptoms, stop flare-ups, and maintain organ function. The varied pharmacological toolbox consists of corticosteroids, immunosuppressants, disease-modifying antirheumatic medications (DMARDs), and nonsteroidal anti-inflammatory drugs (NSAIDs).

Recognizing the unique targets and possible side effects of each medication is essential to understanding its function. For example, NSAIDs treat pain and inflammation, whereas DMARDs alter the immune system's reaction. Strong anti-inflammatory drugs called corticosteroids are frequently used during flare-ups, but because of their long-term side effects, they must be used with caution.

2. Immunomodulatory Treatments

A new frontier in the treatment of lupus is immunomodulatory therapies, which provide focused methods to alter the underlying immune dysregulation. Among the new treatments with promise for the treatment of lupus are biologics, which specifically target immune system components. Examining these treatments' mechanisms of action and the ongoing studies guiding their incorporation into lupus care are essential to comprehending their potential.

3. Corticosteroids: Their Function

Steroids, or corticosteroids, are used to treat lupus in two ways. They have strong anti-inflammatory properties during acute flares, which quickly reduce symptoms. However, a number of negative effects, such as weight gain, increased susceptibility to infections, and bone loss, are linked to their long-term use. In the treatment of lupus, weighing the advantages and disadvantages of corticosteroids becomes essential.

Comprehensive Methods for Lupus Treatment

Beyond pharmaceuticals, holistic approaches acknowledge the connection between mental, emotional, and physical health. Complementary therapies like yoga, acupuncture, and herbal supplements are incorporated into integrative medicine to improve overall wellness. Support for mental health becomes essential, recognizing the emotional cost of having a chronic illness and offering coping mechanisms.

Being aware of the various treatment modalities enables people to take an active role in their care. The treatment plan turns into a cooperative project with shared decision-making at its heart, involving patients and medical professionals. People can modify their treatment plans to suit their individual needs and preferences by realizing the potential of holistic and pharmaceutical interventions.

New Therapies and Clinical Research

1. Positive Advances in Lupus Studies

Research on lupus is characterized by ongoing developments and discoveries. Current research endeavors investigate new therapeutic targets, inventive treatment modalities, and customized approaches to managing lupus. Examining the exciting advancements influencing the direction of lupus treatment in the future is essential to comprehending the current status of lupus research.

2. Taking Part in Clinical Trials

A vital way for people to both access state-of-the-art treatments and further the field of lupus research is through clinical trials. Recognizing the importance of clinical trials entails appreciating how they contribute to improving treatment options, enhancing diagnostic methodologies, and ultimately raising the standard of care for lupus patients.

3. Encouraging By Information

Information is a powerful instrument for enabling lupus patients and their carers. A sense of agency is fostered by an understanding of the many aspects of the disease, including its types and manifestations as well as the complex interactions between environmental and genetic factors. Active involvement in the diagnosis process, cooperative interaction with medical professionals, and well-informed treatment option selection are all components of empowerment.

To sum up, this chapter helps readers navigate the complexities of lupus by acting as a compass. The journey through lupus is complex, involving everything from figuring out the various types and manifestations of the disease to comprehending the genetic and environmental factors at play. Gaining insight into the diagnosis procedure, the functions of different medical specialists, and the range of treatment modalities becomes essential for enabling people to navigate the terrain of lupus with resilience and comprehension. The main objective is still to empower those affected by lupus and the communities around them, encouraging a sense of hope and agency in the face of this complex autoimmune disease, even as we investigate the new areas of lupus research and the possibilities presented by clinical trials.

CHAPTER TWO

Medical Diagnostics and

Perspectives

Handling the Complicated Maze of Lupus

Identification and Management

Making a diagnosis of lupus is like trying to solve a complex puzzle with components that are as different as the illness's symptoms. This chapter provides a roadmap across the complex terrain of lupus diagnosis, including the diagnostic standards, the range of tests that go into a thorough evaluation, and the cooperative efforts of healthcare providers participating in the continuum of care.

Testing and Diagnostic Criteria

Making a diagnosis of lupus requires a sophisticated grasp of the various ways the disease might present itself. It is not a one-size-fits-all process. Often known as the "eleven criteria," the American College of Rheumatology (ACR) criteria offer a uniform framework for lupus diagnosis. The presence of at least four of the eleven criteria—which include a range of clinical and laboratory manifestations—is necessary for a definitive diagnosis.

Still, the diagnostic process goes beyond a to-do list. Because lupus can mirror other disorders, it can be difficult to diagnose it quickly and accurately. Furthermore, the way symptoms change over time may cause a delay in diagnosis, which highlights the importance of constant watchfulness and a comprehensive method of interpreting symptoms.

Laboratory testing are essential in the diagnosis of lupus, providing important pieces of the puzzle. An evaluation for lupus known as antinuclear antibody (ANA) testing looks for antibodies that attack the body's own cells, a characteristic of many autoimmune disorders. Anti-dsDNA, anti-Smith, and anti-phospholipid antibodies are examples of complementary tests that help identify particular lupus subtypes and related problems by fine-tuning the diagnostic procedure.

When musculoskeletal or renal symptoms are suspected, diagnostic imaging techniques like magnetic resonance imaging (MRI) and ultrasound can be used to visualize organ involvement. The amalgamation of different diagnostic modalities aids in a thorough evaluation, directing medical practitioners towards a precise diagnosis and customized measures.

Healthcare Providers Associated with Lupus Management

A collaborative and multidisciplinary strategy is necessary to navigate the complex world of lupus care, utilizing the knowledge and skills of multiple medical specialists. As specialists in autoimmune diseases, rheumatologists frequently lead the diagnosis procedure. Their crucial role in lupus care stems from their comprehension of changing therapy paradigms and their ability to interpret the subtleties of lupus symptoms.

In patients with cutaneous lupus, dermatologists are essential because they use their training to identify dermatological symptoms and provide specific treatments. When renal involvement is evident, nephrologists work together to treat the intricacies of lupus nephritis, a dangerous condition that needs medical intervention only.

As gatekeepers, primary care doctors identify early signs and expedite referrals to specialists. Primary care is incorporated into the lupus care continuum to guarantee a comprehensive strategy that addresses overall health and wellness in addition to lupus-specific issues.

Nurse practitioners and physician assistants play a vital role in the management of lupus patients by offering continuous assistance, education, and care coordination. Because they are easily accessible, patients and providers can develop close relationships that enable lupus patients to take an active role in their care.

When it comes to treating the psychological and emotional effects of having a chronic illness, mental health specialists like psychologists and psychiatrists are essential. Since mental health and physical health are closely related, including mental health specialists in the care team is important because lupus has a significant effect on mental health.

These varied professions work together to provide continuous management and assistance in addition to diagnosis. The cornerstones of successful lupus care include patient-centered care, provider communication, and routine follow-ups, which guarantee that patients receive comprehensive and well-coordinated assistance throughout their journey.

Overview of Treatment Approaches

After piecing together the complex picture of a lupus diagnosis, attention turns to creating a customized treatment strategy. Lupus management is a multidimensional endeavor that takes into account the individual's special demands as well as the disease's specific manifestations. It is not a one-dimensional endeavor.

Immunosuppressive drugs are often the cornerstone of lupus treatment. These drugs, which include mycophenolate mofetil, methotrexate, and hydroxychloroquine, work by modifying the immune system and reducing the inflammatory response that accompanies lupus. The exact symptoms and severity of the disease determine which treatments are best, and a tailored strategy is essential to maximize benefits and reduce adverse effects.

Prednisone is one example of a corticosteroid that is essential for controlling lupus flare-ups because of its quick anti-inflammatory effects. They do, however, have possible adverse effects when used long-term, which emphasizes the careful balancing act between symptom management and reducing medication-related risks.

In the treatment of lupus, biologic therapies—such as belimumab and rituximab—represent a more recent development. By focusing on particular immune system components, these drugs allow for more focused therapies and may lessen the need for broad-spectrum immunosuppression.

A vital part of lupus management goes beyond medication interventions and includes lifestyle changes. In addition to improving general well-being, customized exercise programs, stress reduction techniques, and dietary choices can influence how a disease progresses. Complementary therapies and other holistic techniques, like mindfulness, support traditional treatments and promote a holistic approach to managing lupus.

Because lupus therapy is so complex, people with the disease and their healthcare providers need to communicate frequently. As a guiding concept, shared decision-making enables people to actively engage in choices about their care. A dynamic and adaptable approach to lupus care involves regular monitoring, modifications to treatment programs, and open communication.

This chapter seeks to shed light on the diagnostic nuances, highlight the teamwork of medical professionals, and give an overview of the various treatment modalities that are the cornerstone of the lupus care continuum as we go deeper into the field of lupus care. The path with lupus, characterized by its complexity and uniqueness, calls for a shared commitment to promoting optimal health and well-being in addition to clinical skill and empathy and understanding.

The Patient's Part in the Management of Lupus

The person with lupus becomes crucial in the midst of the complexity of lupus care. Achieving the best results requires empowering people to actively participate in their health journey. Comprehending the subtleties of one's symptoms, taking recommended drugs, and making lifestyle changes become joint efforts between lupus patients and medical professionals.

Educating for Empowerment

An essential component of equipping people to successfully negotiate the maze of lupus is education. Giving them information about the illness, symptoms, and available treatments encourages them to make well-informed decisions. In addition to dispelling misconceptions about lupus, education fosters a sense of agency in patients, empowering them to actively engage in conversations regarding their care.

Patient education is not limited to the clinical setting; it also includes everyday living skills. People take an active role in their treatment, from realizing the value of sun protection to negotiating possible drug side effects, all of which contribute to a common commitment to health and wellbeing.

Developing Coping Mechanisms and Resilience

Resilience is a necessary skill for people with lupus to have in order to overcome the obstacles the disease presents. This chapter explores the methods that people might use to develop resilience. Through the investigation of coping methods for symptom flare-ups and the adoption of a positive outlook, the goal is to enable people living with lupus to confront the challenges of their health journey with courage.

The care of a person with lupus is closely linked to their emotional well-being. Emotional difficulties associated with chronic illness might include everything from anxiety and sadness to the complexities of adjusting to a life altered by the demands of controlling lupus. Professionals in the field of mental health are essential in offering assistance and resources for navigating these emotional terrains.

Including Lifestyle Adjustments

Adjusting one's lifestyle can be one of the most effective ways to treat lupus outside of medication. Dietary factors influence general health, such as following lupus-friendly diets and practicing mindful nutrition. This chapter sheds light on how diet affects lupus and offers helpful advice so that people can make decisions that support their health objectives.

Exercise that is customized to each person's requirements and ability is essential for fostering physical well-being. This investigation attempts to inspire people to take a holistic approach to their health by covering topics such as the value of getting regular movement into daily life and how to modify exercise regimens to account for the swings in energy that sometimes accompany lupus problems.

Handling the Flare and Remission Dynamics

The dynamics of flares and remissions are essential to understanding the lupus journey. This section goes into great detail about how to recognize flare triggers, comprehend the subtleties of emergency action plans during flares, and create plans for staying in remission. A proactive approach and tenacity in adjusting to the ups and downs of symptoms are essential for navigating the uncertain landscape of lupus.

The Emergency Action Plan (EAP), which outlines actions to be performed to lessen the impact of symptoms during flares, turns into a tailored roadmap.

Comprehending the distinct triggers that each person possesses enables preventive actions, which ultimately contribute to efficient flare management. Maintaining remission techniques, such as continuing contact with medical professionals and following treatment regimens, are essential components in promoting long-term stability.

Coping with Lupus: Useful Advice

Creating a strong support network is essential to figuring out the day-to-day logistics of having lupus. This chapter provides guidance on building a support system, encouraging candid communication with family members, and with the emotional difficulties that frequently come with living with a chronic illness.

The complex dance of relationships—both personal and professional—is examined with an emphasis on striking a balance between independence and dependency on other people. Encouraging advice on how to deal with problems at work, maintain a sense of normalcy in daily life, and effectively communicate with healthcare providers all add to the empowerment of people living with lupus.

The joint efforts of healthcare practitioners, lupus patients, and their support networks become evident as we go further into the core of lupus management. This chapter aims to shed light on the complicated nature of lupus care, acknowledging that professional skill alone is not enough to achieve optimal health outcomes; a shared commitment to navigate the difficulties of lupus as a team is also necessary.

CHAPTER THREE

Pharmaceutical Interventions

The complex autoimmune illness lupus necessitates a multimodal approach to treatment. For people with lupus, pharmacological treatments are essential for reducing symptoms, averting flare-ups, and enhancing general quality of life. This chapter delves into the wide range of drugs used in the treatment of lupus, examining their functions, advantages, and possible drawbacks.

Drugs for the Management of Lupus

1. Antimalarial Medication
Antimalarial medications, such chloroquine and hydroxychloroquine, are essential to the treatment of lupus. These drugs help prevent flare-ups of lupus in

addition to managing symptoms related to the skin and joints. Antimalarial medications are useful in treating the chronic form of the disease because of their anti-inflammatory characteristics.

2. NSAIDs, or nonsteroidal anti-inflammatory drugs, NSAIDs, such as naproxen and ibuprofen, are frequently used to treat lupus discomfort and inflammation. Although they alleviate pain in the joints and muscles, their use should be done so with caution because they may have adverse effects, especially on the gastrointestinal tract.

3. Corticosteroids
Strong anti-inflammatory drugs called corticosteroids, including prednisone, are used to fast stop lupus flare-ups. Prolonged use can have negative effects, including as weight gain, increased susceptibility to infections, and bone loss, despite its efficacy. Modifications in dosage and attentive observation are necessary to reduce these dangers.

4. Immunomodulatory Treatments

5. Antirheumatic medications that modify disease (DMARDs)
DMARDs, which target the immune system, include methotrexate and azathioprine, and are intended to alter the course of lupus. These drugs have the ability to

change the course of the disease and are especially helpful when there is significant organ involvement. It is essential to regularly evaluate blood parameters to guarantee their safe and efficient use.

6. biological treatments
In the treatment of lupus, biologic therapies—such as belimumab and rituximab—represent a more recent development. Compared to conventional immunosuppressants, these medications provide a more focused approach by targeting particular immune system components. Their debut is a major step forward, particularly for those who experience refractory lupus signs.

7. Inhibitors of Janus Kinase (JAK)
JAK inhibitors, such as tofacitinib, block particular immune response-related signaling pathways. These drugs have the potential to treat lupus by reducing the hyperactivity of the immune system. Research on their safety and efficacy in various lupus groups is still ongoing.

Corticosteroids: Their Function

1. Use in the Short- and Long-Term

During lupus flares, corticosteroids provide quick relief, but prolonged usage requires cautious thought. Acute symptoms can be successfully controlled with short-term, high-dose regimens; however, long-term usage of steroids may result in problems. In order to prescribe the least amount of medication for the shortest amount of time, doctors try to find a balance.

2. Corticosteroids topical
Topical corticosteroids are used to treat localized skin conditions. Their use efficiently addresses lupus symptoms relating to the skin while minimizing systemic negative effects. In order to maximize results, dermatologists frequently use these medicines into therapy regimens.

3. Injectable Intra-Articular Steroids
Intra-articular steroid injections offer specific treatment for patients with affected joints. These injections, which are injected directly into the afflicted joints, reduce pain and inflammation while improving joint function. Because of their limited nature, there is less chance of systemic exposure and hence fewer adverse consequences.

1. Tailored Treatment Strategies
In lupus care, developing individualized treatment strategies is crucial. A customized strategy is required due to each patient's distinct clinical profile, comorbidities, and preferences. Together with other experts, rheumatologists work to maximize the treatment benefits and minimize any possible adverse effects.

2. Observation and Modifications
It is essential to regularly check lupus patients taking pharmaceutical therapy. Clinical evaluations, imaging examinations, and blood tests are used to measure therapy effectiveness and identify any new issues. Optimal disease control is ensured by timely modifications to drug schedules.

3. Cooperative Decision-Making
People with lupus can take an active role in their treatment by collaborating with healthcare practitioners to make informed decisions together. A collaborative approach to managing the disease is fostered by open conversation regarding pharmaceutical alternatives, potential side effects, and lifestyle factors.

The Changing Face of Medicines for Lupus

1. Individualized Medical Care
Progress in pharmacogenomics has ushered in a period of customized lupus treatment. Clinicians choose medications based on the unique profiles of each patient, taking into account genetic characteristics that affect drug metabolism and reaction. By using a precision approach, side effects are reduced and therapeutic efficacy is increased.

2. Putting New Pathways in Focus
Novel therapeutic targets and therapy approaches for lupus are being investigated by ongoing research. Finding particular immune system elements and signaling pathways can lead to the development of drugs with improved selectivity and fewer side effects.

3. Research Focused on Patients
Patient viewpoints are becoming more and more important in lupus research. Comprehending the effects of drugs on day-to-day functioning, taking into account patient-reported results, and attending to quality of life issues enhance the body of research and lead to more comprehensive therapeutic strategies.

In summary

Pharmacological treatments represent a dynamic and growing element of lupus care. From time-tested antimalarials to cutting-edge biologic medicines, the arsenal against lupus continues to develop. The difficult balance between treatment advantages and potential hazards highlights the significance of tailored, patient-centered care. As researchers unearth new insights and breakthroughs, the quest towards more effective and customized lupus therapies unfolds, bringing hope for improved outcomes and enhanced quality of life for patients living with this complex autoimmune disorder.

CHAPTER FOUR

Emerging Treatments and Clinical

Trials

The landscape of lupus research is dynamic, distinguished by ongoing investigation and innovation. In this chapter, we dig into the intriguing field of new medicines and the relevance of clinical trials in enhancing lupus care.

Promising Developments in Lupus Research

1.Targeted Therapies

Advancements in our understanding of the immune system have paved the road for targeted treatments in lupus treatment. These medicines focus on specific components of the immune system, offering a more targeted approach compared to standard immunosuppressants. In particular, B-cell targeted treatments, such as rituximab, have showed promise in controlling lupus symptoms.

2. Interferon Inhibition
Interferons, signaling proteins that play a role in the immunological response, are commonly hyperactive in lupus. Inhibiting interferon pathways is a burgeoning topic of research. New drugs designed to suppress interferon signals attempt to control the immune system's hyperactivity, providing a novel path for therapeutic intervention.

3.Complement Inhibition
The complement system, a component of the immune system, is implicated in lupus development. Drugs targeting individual components of the complement cascade are under research. Inhibiting complement activation offers potential in minimizing inflammatory damage and moderating lupus symptoms.

Participating in Clinical Trials

1. The Importance of Clinical Trials
Clinical trials are crucial in testing the safety and efficacy of new lupus therapies. Participation in clinical trials not only allows individuals access to cutting-edge medicines but also contributes to the collective knowledge advancing lupus care. Rigorous scientific research in clinical trials forms the foundation for evidence-based treatment options.

2. Informed Decision-Making
Individuals seeking involvement in clinical trials are encouraged to engage in informed decision-making. Understanding the trial's aims, potential risks, and rewards is vital. Informed consent methods give full information, permitting participants to make decisions consistent with their beliefs and health goals.

Phases of Clinical Trials

Clinical studies continue through several phases, each serving a specific purpose

1. Phase I
Primarily focused on safety, Phase I trials contain a small number of participants. Researchers analyze how the

new therapy interacts with the body and detect potential negative effects.

2. Phase II
Building on safety data, Phase II trials extend participant numbers to examine the treatment's effectiveness. Researchers attempt to establish the ideal dosage and further assess safety.

3. Phase III
Phase III trials use bigger participant groups to confirm efficacy and monitor negative effects in varied populations. Results from Phase III trials affect regulatory decisions on drug approval.

4. Phase IV
Post-approval, Phase IV trials continue to examine a treatment's long-term safety and effectiveness in real-world situations.

Access to Experimental Treatments

Access to experimental medicines through clinical trials is a rare option for patients with lupus. Investigational drugs may give alternate possibilities when regular treatments prove ineffective. Collaboration between healthcare practitioners, researchers, and participants enables full support throughout the trial process.

Overcoming Barriers to Participation

While clinical trials offer enormous potential, various impediments to participation exist. Geographic limits, lack of information, and concerns about potential adverse effects are common hurdles. Initiatives to alleviate these hurdles include improving public awareness, developing collaboration amongst research centers, and introducing steps to promote accessibility.

Bridging the Gap: Translational Research

1. Translating Bench Discoveries to Bedside Care
Translational research bridges the gap between laboratory findings and clinical applications. Insights acquired from understanding lupus at the molecular and cellular levels inform the development of innovative therapeutics. The translation of bench research to bedside care accelerates the availability of novel medications for persons with lupus.

2. Biomarkers and Personalized Medicine
Advancements in translational research contribute to the identification of biomarkers — measurable indications of disease activity. Biomarkers aid in predicting therapy responses and adapting interventions

to particular patient profiles. The era of customized medicine in lupus is complemented by translational studies that refine treatment options based on specific biological markers.

3. Navigating the Clinical Trial Journey

4. Patient Advocacy and Support
Patient advocacy organizations play a critical role in aiding persons navigate the clinical trial path. These organizations provide resources, educational materials, and forums for sharing experiences. Empowering patients with information develops a sense of community and resilience throughout the trial process.

5. Comprehensive Informed Consent
Informed consent is a cornerstone of ethical clinical research. Ensuring that participants completely know the trial's aims, potential risks, and benefits encourages transparency and confidence. Clear communication between researchers and participants builds a foundation for a collaborative and ethical research environment.

6. Ethical Considerations in Clinical Trials
Ethical considerations are crucial in lupus clinical studies. Safeguarding participant rights, maintaining confidentiality, and upholding scientific integrity are key values. Ethical conduct in research not only respects the

autonomy and well-being of participants but also contributes to the credibility and dependability of trial outcomes.

- The Future Landscape of Lupus Care

1. Personalized Treatment Algorithms
As translational research and clinical trials continue, the future landscape of lupus care holds the potential of tailored therapy algorithms. Tailoring therapies based on individual patient features, genetics, and biomarkers will maximize therapy success while avoiding unwanted effects.

2. Collaborative Research Networks
The formation of collaborative research networks generates synergies among scholars, institutions, and industry partners. These networks promote large-scale clinical trials, enabling the examination of multiple treatment techniques and therapies. Collaborative efforts speed the translation of research findings into actual improvements in lupus care.

3. Patient-Centric Outcomes
The future of lupus care promotes patient-centric outcomes. Integrating patient-reported outcomes into clinical trial assessments provides vital insights into the influence of therapies on daily life, functioning, and general well-being. Recognizing the holistic components

of health contributes to more complete and patient-centered care.

In summary

Emerging medicines and clinical trials are the vanguard of lupus research, bringing hope for expanded therapy options and improved outcomes. The united efforts of academics, healthcare professionals, and persons with lupus move the field forward, underlining the necessity of active engagement in clinical research. As we traverse the expanding terrain of lupus care, the pursuit of breakthrough treatments and the commitment to patient-centered research establish the framework for a future where effective, tailored, and accessible interventions redefine the standard of lupus care.

CHAPTER FIVE

Holistic Approaches to Lupus

Management

Lupus, a complex autoimmune disorder, demands a varied approach to management. In this chapter, we look into holistic solutions that expand beyond conventional medical treatments, investigating integrative medicine and alternative therapies, as well as addressing the critical component of mental health assistance for persons navigating the problems of lupus.

Integrative Medicine and Alternative Therapies

1. Mind-Body Practices: Integrative medicine stresses the relationship between mind and body. Practices such as yoga, meditation, and tai chi offer not just physical advantages but also contribute to stress reduction. Mindfulness methods can equip individuals to manage the psychological toll of living with lupus.

2. Acupuncture and Traditional Chinese Medicine: Acupuncture, founded in traditional Chinese medicine, has earned recognition for relieving pain and inflammation in lupus patients. Herbal medicines, as part of holistic techniques, are researched for their possible advantages in conjunction with medical therapies.

3. Massage and Physical Therapies: Massage treatment can provide relief from muscle and joint pain associated with lupus. Additionally, physical therapy tailored to individual needs help to greater flexibility and overall well-being.

Mental Health Support for Lupus Patients

1. Psychological Counseling: The emotional burden of chronic illness is important. Professional counseling gives a safe space for people and families to negotiate

the emotional problems associated with lupus, strengthening coping mechanisms and resilience.

2. Support Groups and Peer Networks: Uniting with others who have similar problems can be useful. Support groups and online communities give a platform for individuals to share thoughts, seek guidance, and find solace in a community that knows the subtleties of life with lupus.

3. Cognitive Behavioral Therapy (CBT): CBT is a therapeutic method that helps patients reframe negative thought patterns and create effective coping mechanisms. In the setting of lupus, CBT can benefit in controlling stress, anxiety, and depression.

Balancing Holistic Approaches with Medical Care

1. Collaboration with Healthcare Providers: Integrative and alternative therapies should complement, not replace, traditional medical care. Open communication with healthcare providers is vital to maintain a cohesive and safe approach to comprehensive lupus management.

2. Personalized Treatment Plans: Recognizing the particular nature of lupus, holistic methods should be adapted to each person's specific needs. Personalized treatment strategies address criteria such as overall health, unique lupus manifestations, and individual preferences.

3. Safety and Evidence-Based Practices:
   While exploring alternative remedies, it's vital to prioritize safety. Consultation with healthcare specialists ensures that chosen approaches match with evidence-based practices and do not pose hazards or conflicts with prescribed medications.

Empowering Individuals on Their Holistic Journey

1. Education and Resources: Providing comprehensive knowledge on various holistic approaches empowers individuals to make educated judgments. Access to trustworthy information facilitates a fuller grasp of the potential benefits and limitations of each technique.

2. Incorporating Holistic Practices into Daily Life: Holistic techniques are most effective when smoothly integrated into daily activities. Practical recommendations on implementing mindfulness, dietary adjustments, and therapeutic activities boost their accessibility for those with lupus.

3. Measuring Progress and Adjusting Approaches: Regular assessments of holistic practices allow individuals to quantify their influence on lupus symptoms. Flexibility in altering techniques ensures that the holistic journey matches with evolving demands and the dynamic nature of lupus.

CHAPTER SIX

Nutrition and Diet

In order to effectively manage this complicated autoimmune disease, it is essential to comprehend the complex interaction between nutrition and lupus. This chapter explores the complex field of nutrition, including how diet choices affect lupus symptoms, what constitutes a lupus-friendly diet, and the function of dietary supplements.

The Role of Nutrition in the Management and Treatment of Lupus

Given that lupus is characterized by immune system malfunction and persistent inflammation, it is important to examine the role that nutrition plays in the course of the disease. In people with lupus, dietary decisions can have a major influence on inflammation levels, the intensity of symptoms, and general well-being.

Anti-Inflammatory Foods and Inflammation:

One characteristic of lupus is chronic inflammation. Some foods may be able to reduce inflammation because of their anti-inflammatory qualities, according to research. Including foods high in omega-3 fatty acids, such walnuts, flaxseeds, and fatty fish, may help control inflammation. Likewise, vibrant fruits and vegetables—especially those rich in antioxidants—contribute to a diet that reduces inflammation.

Managing Nutrient Consumption:

Sustaining an optimally balanced diet is crucial for those suffering from lupus. Enough consumption of vital nutrients, such as vitamins, minerals, and antioxidants, promotes general well-being and strengthens the immune system. Having a colorful and varied plate can aid in obtaining the wide range of nutrients required for optimum performance.

Food Sensitivities' Effects

Certain foods may cause hypersensitivity in certain lupus patients, which can exacerbate their symptoms. Finding and treating these sensitivity through a food diary or elimination diet can help reduce symptoms and enhance quality of life.

Diets & Meal Planning for People with Lupus

Dietary modifications made in accordance with lupus-friendly guidelines can improve general health and symptom management. A number of dietary strategies have drawn interest due to their possible advantages when it comes to lupus.

The Mediterranean Diet

The Mediterranean diet places a strong emphasis on whole grains, fruits, vegetables, lean proteins, and healthy fats, especially olive oil. It is modeled after the customary eating habits of the nations that border the Mediterranean Sea. This diet may help control lupus symptoms since it is high in anti-inflammatory and antioxidant substances.

Plant-Based Diets:

Diets based on plants, such as vegetarian and vegan regimens, have been studied for their anti-inflammatory properties. These diets emphasize nutrient- and fiber-dense plant-based foods such fruits, vegetables, legumes, and nuts. But to guarantee sufficient consumption of important nutrients like protein, iron, and vitamin B12, careful preparation is necessary.

Options Free of Dairy and Gluten:

Some lupus sufferers may experience symptom alleviation by switching to a diet devoid of dairy or gluten. Gluten, which can be present in dairy products, wheat, and other grains, might make certain people irritated or sensitive. When putting these dietary changes into practice, it is important to look into other sources of these vital minerals.

Nutritional Add-ons and Their Advantages

In managing lupus, supplements might be helpful in adding extra support to dietary requirements. But it's crucial to take supplements cautiously and under medical professionals' supervision.

Supplementing with vitamins and minerals:

The immune system and general health are significantly impacted by specific vitamins and minerals. For example, vitamin D deficiency is common in lupus patients and is necessary for immunological modulation. Anti-inflammatory properties are partially attributed to omega-3 fatty acids. Comprehending the distinct requirements and possible inadequacies of lupus patients facilitates the customization of supplementation schemes.

Supplements with Herbs:

The possible anti-inflammatory effects of herbal supplements, like those containing ginger and turmeric, are being studied. The potential of turmeric, which contains curcumin, to alter inflammatory pathways has been investigated. Despite its potential, people should use prudence and speak with medical professionals because herbal supplements may have contraindications or interfere with pharmaceuticals.

Gut Health and Probiotics:

Research on the relationship between autoimmune diseases and intestinal health is only getting started. Beneficial bacteria called probiotics contribute to the upkeep of a balanced gut microbiome. Immunological system performance and general well-being may benefit from gut health support.

Educating People About Nutrition to Empower Them

Professionals in Healthcare Offering Nutritional Advice:

Nutritional advice is individualized and supported by evidence when healthcare professionals and registered dietitians work together. Dietary advice are customized based on individual health profiles, medication interactions, and unique indications of lupus.

Tips for Meal Planning and Preparation:

It's crucial to have realistic methods for grocery shopping, meal planning, and cooking lupus-friendly meals. These suggestions consider the difficulties that lupus sufferers could have on a regular basis, such as joint pain or exhaustion.

Managing Eating's Social and Cultural Aspects:

Changes in diet can have an effect on the social and cultural aspects of eating. Techniques for handling dietary constraints in social situations and customizing lupus-friendly options to cultural tastes enable people to uphold their nutritional objectives in a variety of situations.

Providing Sustainable and Pleasurable Eating Habits

Steer clear of restrictive mindsets:

Promoting a healthy, pleasurable, and balanced attitude toward food is essential. Maintaining a healthy connection with food and avoiding unduly restrictive diets are important for long-term sustainability and general wellbeing.

Keeping an eye on and modifying dietary plans:

People can make educated dietary changes when they regularly evaluate their food choices and how they affect their lupus symptoms. It is ensured that dietary regimens are flexible enough to respond to changing lifestyle requirements and changing health needs.

Including Variety and Tastes:

Stressing the value of varied and tasty meals improves the taste experience in general. The nutritional journey is made more exciting and varied by experimenting with various cuisines and recipes that follow lupus-friendly guidelines.

The Changing Field of Nutritional Studies in Lupus

Trends in Current Research:

Our knowledge of the relationship between lupus and nutrition is constantly being improved by ongoing study. Readers receive the most recent information via updates on research that have been conducted recently that examine the effects of particular dietary components and how they affect lupus symptoms.

Personalized Nutrition and Nutrigenomics:

The science of nutrigenomics, which examines how a person's genetic composition affects how they respond to foods, is rapidly developing. There is potential for improving results and customizing dietary advice by investigating personalized nutrition based on genetic characteristics.

Possible Innovations in the Future:

Potential discoveries in the molecular processes relating food to lupus may arise as nutritional science progresses.

Following these advancements gives hope for creative methods of controlling and possibly preventing symptoms associated with lupus.

Overcoming Obstacles and Difficulties

Resolving Nutritional Inequalities:

It is imperative to recognize and resolve inequalities in the availability of wholesome food. Techniques for getting beyond obstacles related to finances, location, or culture to acquire and incorporate wholesome food options into everyday life are covered.

Handling Perplexity About Diet:

It can be intimidating to see so much information available about diets and supplements. Dispelling popular myths and giving people the means to assess nutritional advice critically enable people to make sense of the frequently bewildering world of dietary knowledge.

Working Together to Make Decisions with Healthcare Providers:

It is stressed that medical professionals have a crucial role in advising patients on diet. Promoting transparent communication and cooperative decision-making guarantees that people with lupus have all-encompassing and well-coordinated support for their dietary journey.

Beyond Nutrition: Dietary Practices and Hydration

Water Content and Its Effects:

A vital component of general health is being properly hydrated. In order to promote holistic well-being, it is essential to investigate the significance of hydration in lupus therapy, including its possible effects on joint health and organ function.

Conscious Eating Techniques:

Being present and focused during meals is part of mindful eating. Including mindful eating practices can improve eating experiences in general, encourage better digestion, and foster a healthy connection with food.

Harmonizing Nutrient Density with Indulgences:

It's crucial to strike a balance between indulging in rare occasions and eating a diet rich in nutrients. There is discussion on how to incorporate goodies and make thoughtful decisions without sacrificing overall nutritional objectives. This harmony makes sure people can enjoy food and maintain good health at the same time.

Participation in the Community and Peer Assistance

Programs for Community Nutrition:

Participating in community-based nutrition programs helps to create a supportive atmosphere for lupus patients. These initiatives support a sense of community and general well-being by providing information, resources, and chances for shared activities. Having access to community projects gives people a forum on which to discuss, share, and celebrate their accomplishments.

Nutrition Initiatives Led by Peers:

Initiatives spearheaded by people who have successfully navigated their own dietary issues while living with lupus use the strength of peer support to offer support, encouragement, and a feeling of community. Peer-led programs foster a community in which people may support one another on their nutritional journeys, relate to one other's experiences, and exchange advice.

Recipe sharing and interactive platforms:

By utilizing internet forums, nutrition advice, and interactive conversation to share recipes, people can develop a virtual community where they can share ideas, encourage one another, and celebrate their nutritional accomplishments. Online resources make it possible for people to stay in touch, even when they live far apart, which promotes a sense of community among those who are interested in nutrition.

Prospective Aspects and Ongoing Education

Keeping Up with Nutritional Research:

Stressing the value of keeping up with current findings and developments in the field of nutrition science guarantees that people are able to modify their dietary plans in response to new information. Being up to date on the most recent research in the dynamic field of nutrition enables people to make well-informed dietary decisions.

Including New Research in Everyday Activities:

Giving advice on how people can actually incorporate changing dietary recommendations into their daily lives as new research becomes available guarantees that the knowledge gathered from continuing study is translated into practical actions. By taking the initiative, people can adjust their diet according to the most recent research, which fosters ongoing progress in the treatment of lupus.

Promoting a Healthful Connection with Food:

In closing, the chapter emphasizes how important it is to develop a healthy relationship with food. People with lupus can start a path that improves their entire quality of life and physical well-being by adopting a holistic, balanced, and customized approach to eating.

In summary

An extensive examination of nutrition and diet in relation to managing lupus is provided in Chapter 7. This chapter gives people useful information and doable solutions, including topics such as how nutrition affects inflammation, lupus-friendly diets, nutritional supplements, and overcoming obstacles.

When people are knowledgeable about how nutrition affects lupus, they can make decisions that will improve their health. People with lupus may confidently and resiliently negotiate the complex world of nutrition by developing a healthy relationship with food, connecting with supporting communities, and staying up to date on new findings.

This chapter offers a basis for people to adjust and incorporate new information into their dietary practices as our awareness of the relationship between nutrition and lupus deepens. In the end, a customized and all-encompassing approach to diet becomes an essential part of a comprehensive plan for improving general health and treating lupus.

CHAPTER SEVEN

Physical fitness and well-being

We examine the critical role that exercise plays in the overall management of lupus in this chapter. We explore the many facets of sustaining physical well-being in the setting of lupus, from realizing the significance of exercise for lupus patients to customizing exercise regimens and introducing moderate activities into everyday life.

Exercise Is Crucial for People with Lupus

1. Handling Joint Pain and Fatigue:
Frequent exercise has been demonstrated to reduce joint pain and weariness, two frequent lupus symptoms. Appropriate physical activity contributes to a better

overall sense of wellbeing by preserving joint flexibility and reducing muscular tightness.

2. Improving Heart Health:
People with lupus are concerned about cardiovascular consequences. By increasing cardiovascular fitness, lowering the risk of cardiovascular problems, and enhancing circulation, exercise—especially aerobic exercise—promotes heart health.

3. Encouraging Mental Wellness:
Patients with lupus should especially benefit from exercise's positive effects on mental health. The body's natural mood enhancers, endorphins, are released when you exercise, and they can help reduce stress, worry, and depression that are frequently linked to long-term conditions like lupus.

Customizing Exercise to Meet Personal Needs

1. Consultation with Medical Specialists:
It's important for people with lupus to speak with their healthcare provider before starting an exercise program. Healthcare specialists can provide individualized recommendations, considering the individual's overall health, unique lupus manifestations, and any potential limits.

2. Choosing Appropriate Activities:

Not all workouts are suited for everyone with lupus. Low-impact sports such as swimming, walking, or cycling are generally recommended, as they are mild on the joints. Tailoring the type of exercise to individual tastes and capabilities is crucial to long-term commitment.

3. Gradual Progression and Flexibility:
Lupus sufferers should adopt a gradual approach to exercise, enabling the body to adjust. Starting with low-intensity activities and gradually increasing the time and intensity helps prevent overexertion. Flexibility exercises, such as yoga, contribute to joint flexibility and overall well-being.

Incorporating Gentle Activities into Daily Life

1. Everyday Movement and Lifestyle Changes:
Incorporating activity into daily life is vital for lupus patients. Simple actions such as stretching, taking brief walks, or adding movements into daily routines aid to maintaining joint mobility and reducing stiffness.

2. Adaptive Exercise Equipment:
For persons with unique physical limitations, adaptive exercise equipment can be beneficial. This includes equipment designed to accommodate varying mobility

levels and joint ailments, making exercise more accessible and pleasant.

3. Home-Based Exercise Programs:
Developing home-based fitness programs provides flexibility for lupus sufferers. With advice from healthcare specialists or exercise experts, individuals can build routines that suit their interests, accommodate their energy levels, and are adaptive to changing health situations.

Lifestyle Adjustments

1. Stress Management Techniques:
Stress management is crucial to lupus management. Exercise, particularly exercises like yoga or tai chi, not only adds to physical well-being but also functions as an efficient stress management strategy. Incorporating mindful movement activities can help patients cope with the emotional issues connected with lupus.

2. Sleep Hygiene for Lupus Patients:
Quality sleep is vital for those with lupus to manage fatigue and maintain overall health. Regular exercise has been related to increased sleep quality. Establishing consistent sleep patterns and adding modest pre-sleep exercises can lead to better sleep hygiene.

3. Balancing Work, Rest, and Leisure:

Striking a balance between work, rest, and leisure is vital for those with lupus. Tailoring exercise programs to accommodate energy levels, scheduling rest days, and adding fun physical activities into leisure time contribute to a healthy and sustainable lifestyle.

Empowering Individuals Through Exercise Education

1. Educational Resources and Guidance:
Providing educational resources on the benefits of exercise for lupus patients empowers individuals to make educated decisions. Guidance in choosing acceptable activities, understanding the necessity of moderate progression, and recognizing signs of overexertion enhances exercise efficacy and safety.

2. Collaboration with Exercise Professionals:
Collaborating with fitness professionals, such as physical therapists or certified trainers experienced in working with patients with chronic conditions, guarantees individualized coaching. These professionals may build tailored workout plans, monitor progress, and provide continuous assistance.

3. Group Exercise Classes and Supportive Communities:

Participating in group exercise courses geared for individuals with lupus fosters a supportive environment. These programs build camaraderie, inspiration, and a common awareness of the problems faced by participants, boosting the whole workout experience.

Overcoming Exercise Challenges and Adapting Strategies

1. Dealing with Fluctuating Symptoms:
Lupus symptoms might fluctuate, altering energy levels and physical skills. Adapting exercise tactics to suit changes in symptoms, such as lowering intensity or choosing alternate activities during flare-ups, supports continuing involvement with physical activity.

2. Addressing Mobility Limitations:
Some patients with lupus may develop movement problems. Tailoring exercise routines to focus on improving specific areas of mobility or engaging in sitting exercises fosters inclusivity and encourages individuals to work within their physical capabilities.

3. Motivational Strategies and Goal Setting:
Establishing realistic and motivating goals is crucial for maintaining exercise motivation. Setting reasonable

targets, evaluating progress, and recognizing victories, no matter how minor, contribute to a good outlook and ongoing commitment to physical activity.

Future Perspectives on Exercise and Lupus

1. Advancements in Adaptive Technologies:
Ongoing breakthroughs in adaptive technologies provide hope for patients with lupus. Innovations in exercise equipment and technologies customized to diverse physical abilities contribute to make exercise more accessible and pleasurable.

2. Integration with Telehealth:
The integration of exercise programs with telehealth platforms facilitates remote access to guidance and support. Telehealth enables individuals to connect with healthcare professionals or fitness experts from the comfort of their homes, promoting continuity in exercise routines.

3. Research on Exercise and Lupus Outcomes:
Continued research on the outcomes of exercise in lupus management contributes to evolving guidelines and recommendations. Monitoring research developments ensures that individuals can benefit from the latest evidence-based approaches to physical activity.

In summary

Chapter 8 sheds light on the pivotal role of exercise and physical well-being in the holistic management of lupus. From managing symptoms and enhancing cardiovascular health to tailoring exercise to individual needs and incorporating gentle activities into daily life, this chapter provides a comprehensive guide for individuals navigating the complexities of lupus.

Empowered with knowledge about the benefits of exercise, the importance of individualized approaches, and strategies to overcome challenges, individuals with lupus can embark on a journey towards improved physical well-being. As advancements in adaptive technologies and telehealth continue to shape the landscape of exercise interventions, individuals can stay informed and embrace innovative approaches to enhance their overall health and quality of life while living with lupus.

CHAPTER EIGHT

Modifications to Lifestyle

This chapter explores the complex issues surrounding lifestyle modifications for lupus patients. This chapter offers comprehensive insights into navigating the challenges and improving the general well-being of those affected by lupus. These insights range from stress management techniques and sleep hygiene optimization to finding balance in work, rest, and leisure.

Techniques for Stress Management

• 1. Meditation and Mindfulness:
Meditation and other mindfulness techniques are useful tools for stress management. People with lupus can manage the emotional difficulties brought on by the

illness by practicing present-moment awareness and adopting a nonjudgmental attitude. Stress management now requires the use of mindfulness exercises and guided meditation sessions.

2. Breathing Techniques:
You can incorporate deep breathing exercises into your daily routines to help you relax. Methods like progressive muscle relaxation and diaphragmatic breathing ease stress, lessen anxiety, and foster calmness. Regular practice of these exercises equips people to effectively manage stress.

3. Yoga and Mild Stretching:
Yoga, which is well-known for its mind-body connection, has advantages for the body and the mind. Yoga poses and gentle stretching increase flexibility, release tense muscles, and help people feel less stressed. Yoga poses that are customized to each practitioner's abilities guarantee accessibility for people with different levels of physical comfort.

Sleep hygiene in individuals with lupus

1. Creating a Regular Sleep Schedule:
For people with lupus, sleep patterns must be consistent. A regular sleep schedule that includes regular wake-up and bedtimes improves the circadian rhythm of the body.

Establishing a peaceful evening routine informs the body when it's time to relax, resulting in higher-quality sleep.

2. Enhancing the Ambience for Sleep:
Setting up a comfortable sleeping environment is essential for people with lupus. This entails keeping the bedroom quiet, dark, and cool, buying cozy pillows and mattresses, and reducing noise pollution. These modifications help you get a better night's sleep.

3. Reducing Stimulants Just Before Sleep:
People who have lupus should be aware of stimulants that may cause sleep disturbances. Reducing caffeine and nicotine consumption is beneficial for improved sleep hygiene, especially in the evening. Furthermore, limiting the use of electronics before bed reduces the negative effects of blue light on circadian rhythms.

Juggling Work, Play, and Rest

1. Adaptable Work Schedules:
Understanding the particular difficulties that people with lupus encounter, it becomes essential to support flexible work schedules. People can balance their work and health obligations with flexibility thanks to options like remote work, flexible hours, or part-time schedules.

2. Rest Periods on a Schedule:

The importance of striking a balance between activity and rest is recognized when regular rest periods are incorporated into daily schedules. These pauses provide moments of renewal for people with lupus, assisting in the management of fatigue and preventing burnout. Maintaining energy levels requires striking a balance between purposeful rest periods and work-related tasks.

3. Relaxing Recreational Activities:
Relaxation-promoting leisure activities are essential for general wellbeing. People with lupus can relax and rejuvenate through hobbies, artistic endeavors, or time spent in nature. Customizing leisure pursuits to individual interests guarantees that unwinding becomes an essential aspect of everyday existence.

Encouraging People via Work-Life Harmony

1. Realistic Work Expectations Setting:
Maintaining a healthy work-life balance in the workplace requires setting reasonable expectations. People who have lupus should be transparent with their employers regarding their medical needs and work together to establish realistic goals for the workplace. Openness promotes comprehension and permits preemptive adjustments.

2. Establishing a Helpful Workplace:

Fostering a supportive work environment entails designing areas where people with lupus feel accepted and understood. This could entail educating coworkers and managers, implementing policies that assist staff in managing long-term medical conditions, and holding awareness campaigns.

3. Resources for Education on Work-Life Harmony:
By offering educational materials on work-life balance, people with lupus can take charge of their health and manage their professional obligations. Workshops, lectures, and educational resources all support an environment where employees' well-being is valued and a balanced approach to work is encouraged.

Modifications to Lifestyle and Flares of Lupus

1. Identifying Flare Triggers:
Making meaningful lifestyle changes requires an understanding of potential triggers for lupus flares. Common triggers include stress, nutrition, lack of sleep, and overexertion. Lupus sufferers gain from being aware of these triggers and taking preventative action to lessen their effects.

2. Plans of Action for Flare Emergencies:

Creating customized emergency action plans helps people with lupus react to flares in a useful way. These plans might include instructions on when to seek medical attention, contact details for healthcare providers, and detailed steps for managing symptoms. Being ready gives you more confidence when facing difficult times.

3. Techniques for Sustaining Remission:
Modest lifestyle changes are essential for lupus patients to maintain remission. A proactive approach to addressing new symptoms, regular medical check-ups, treatment plan adherence, and continuous stress management are some examples of strategies. Maintaining remission requires cooperation between patients and healthcare professionals, which is ensured by regular communication.

Providing Education on Lifestyles to Empower People

1. Workshops and webinars for education:
Organizing informative webinars and workshops gives lupus sufferers a way to get information about changing their lifestyle. Work-life balance, stress management, good sleep hygiene, and flare-coping techniques are a few possible topics. Interactive meetings encourage participation and provide people the tools they need to make good changes.

2. Peer Assistance Systems:
By creating peer support networks, people with lupus can exchange experiences and knowledge about lifestyle modifications. Peer-led projects build a feeling of community by connecting people who are going through similar things. Peer support offers helpful advice, motivation, and a common understanding of the journey with lupus.

3. Educational Resources That Are Accessible:
Having dependable information available to people with lupus is ensured by the provision of accessible educational materials. These could include booklets, websites, and guides covering different facets of lifestyle modifications. Materials that are easy to read and understand support proactive self-management and well-informed decision-making.

Overcoming Obstacles and Choosing to Be Resilient

1. Taking Care of Workplace Stigma:
It will take activism and education to eradicate the stigma in the workplace related to chronic conditions. It is beneficial for coworkers and employers to comprehend lupus and how it affects people's lives. Sensitivity training, awareness campaigns, and open

discussions all help to create a welcoming and encouraging work atmosphere.

2. Managing Cultural and Social Expectations:
For people with lupus, social and cultural expectations can be difficult. It takes open communication with friends, family, and social circles to navigate these expectations. Establishing boundaries, asking for help, and educating loved ones about the illness all help to create a network that recognizes and meets the needs of each individual.

3. Building Emotional Hardiness:
Developing emotional resilience is essential for managing lifestyle changes brought on by lupus. Resilience is influenced by accepting the illness, getting emotional support when required, and creating coping strategies. Support groups, therapy, and mindfulness exercises are all essential for fostering emotional well-being.

Perspectives for the Future of Lifestyle Modifications in Lupus Management

1. Technological Advancements in Remote Work:
The field of remote work technology is always changing as long as technology keeps getting better.

Advancements in digital collaboration platforms, augmented reality, and adaptable work arrangements augment prospects for people with lupus to engage in the labor force while satisfying their medical requirements. Future work-life balance considerations will prominently feature the seamless integration of remote work.

2. Customized Apps for Stress Management:
Promising developments include the creation of individualized stress management applications for lupus patients. These apps can provide real-time interventions, personalized exercises based on a user's unique triggers, and an understanding of stress patterns through the use of AI algorithms. Technology is being used in stress management in a more customized way that promotes proactive mental health.

3. Programs for Workplace Wellness for Chronic Illnesses:
Subsequent workplace wellness initiatives might include modules tailored to the needs of people with long-term illnesses like lupus. In the workplace, customized tools, training sessions, and support systems all help to foster an environment where employees' health and wellbeing are given top priority. Complete workplace wellness programs become the norm when chronic illness awareness is incorporated.

4. Developments in Sleep Monitoring Technology:

As they advance, sleep tracking gadgets offer increasingly complex insights into the quantity and quality of sleep. In the future, gadgets might provide tailored advice on how to enhance sleep hygiene, adjust to unique circadian cycles, and deal with particular sleep issues related to lupus. Technology plays a crucial role in enabling people to optimize their sleep schedules.

5. Improved Platforms for Peer Assistance:
Peer support platforms will be improved in the future, bringing more dynamic and interactive spaces for people with lupus. AI-powered peer matching systems, gamified challenges, and virtual support groups all help to strengthen bonds between people going through similar life transitions. Peer support platforms are evolving to become essential components of continuous emotional and practical support.

6. Including Cultural Competence in Supporting Materials:
Given the diversity of the lupus community, cultural competence will be a key component of future support materials. The emphasis of educational resources, seminars, and support groups is on appreciating and comprehending the cultural subtleties that could affect changes in way of life. In order to guarantee that support is relevant and available to people from different cultural backgrounds, inclusivity becomes essential.

7. Intersectionality in Lupus Advocacy:
The intersectionality of identities and experiences is addressed in advocacy efforts for lupus patients. Future initiatives work towards dismantling systemic barriers and biases that may disproportionately affect certain groups within the lupus community. The advocacy landscape becomes more nuanced, acknowledging and addressing the unique challenges faced by individuals with intersecting identities.

8. Collaboration with Mental Health Professionals:
The integration of mental health professionals into lupus care teams becomes more commonplace. Collaborative efforts between rheumatologists, primary care physicians, and mental health professionals ensure a comprehensive approach to lifestyle adjustments. Regular mental health check-ins, counseling services, and psychoeducational support contribute to holistic well-being.

Conclusion: Navigating a Balanced and Empowered Life with Lupus

Chapter 9 serves as a comprehensive exploration of lifestyle adjustments for individuals living with lupus.

From managing stress and optimizing sleep hygiene to balancing work, rest, and leisure, this chapter provides a roadmap for navigating the complexities of life with lupus.

As we look toward the future, the landscape of lifestyle adjustments in lupus management continues to evolve, guided by innovations in technology, a deeper understanding of individual needs, and a commitment to fostering inclusivity. The empowerment of individuals with lupus involves not only addressing current challenges but also anticipating and proactively adapting to the changing dynamics of work, relationships, and overall well-being.

By embracing the future perspectives outlined in this chapter, individuals with lupus can navigate their daily lives with resilience, informed decision-making, and a sense of empowerment. The collective efforts of healthcare professionals, advocates, and the broader community contribute to creating an environment where individuals with lupus can lead balanced, fulfilling, and empowered lives.

CHAPTER NINE

Coping with Flares and Remissions

This chapter focuses on the intricate aspects of managing lupus flares and navigating periods of remission. From identifying triggers and developing emergency action plans to strategies for maintaining remission, individuals with lupus and their caregivers gain valuable insights into coping with the dynamic nature of the disease.

Identifying Triggers for Lupus Flares

1. Understanding Individual Triggers:
Lupus flares can be triggered by a variety of factors, and recognizing these individual triggers is a crucial step in proactive management. These triggers may include stress, exposure to sunlight, infections, hormonal changes, and specific medications. By keeping a detailed

symptom journal, individuals can identify patterns and potential triggers unique to their experience.

2. Monitoring Dietary Influences:
Diet plays a role in lupus management, and certain foods may contribute to flare-ups. Monitoring dietary influences, such as identifying potential allergens or inflammatory foods, empowers individuals to make informed choices. Collaboration with a healthcare professional or nutritionist can help create a personalized dietary plan that aligns with lupus management goals.

3. Tracking Emotional and Environmental Factors:
Emotional and environmental factors can significantly impact lupus flares. Stress, anxiety, and exposure to environmental pollutants are common contributors. Utilizing stress-management techniques, practicing mindfulness, and creating a supportive living environment contribute to minimizing the impact of these factors on lupus symptoms.

Emergency Action Plans for Flares

1. Personalized Flare Response Strategies:
Developing personalized flare response strategies involves working closely with healthcare professionals to create a tailored action plan. This plan may include specific steps to address worsening symptoms, adjust

medications, and guidelines on when to seek immediate medical attention. A well-defined plan enhances individuals' ability to navigate flares confidently.

2. Communication with Healthcare Providers:
Effective communication with healthcare providers is paramount during flares. Regular check-ins, reporting changes in symptoms promptly, and collaborating on adjustments to the treatment plan ensure a proactive approach. Healthcare providers become essential partners in managing flares and preventing escalation of symptoms.

3. Incorporating Holistic Approaches:
Holistic approaches, such as integrative medicine and alternative therapies, can complement traditional medical interventions during flares. These may include acupuncture, herbal supplements, or mind-body practices. Collaborating with healthcare professionals ensures that holistic approaches align with overall treatment goals and are integrated into the flare response plan.

Strategies for Remission Maintenance

1. Adherence to Medication Regimens:

Consistent adherence to prescribed medications is fundamental for maintaining remission. Individuals with lupus should work closely with their healthcare team to understand the importance of each medication, potential side effects, and the role each plays in managing the disease. Any concerns or difficulties with medications should be promptly discussed with healthcare providers.

2. Regular Monitoring of Disease Activity:
Regular monitoring of disease activity, including laboratory tests and clinical assessments, aids in early detection of changes that may indicate potential flares. Individuals in remission should maintain regular follow-ups with their healthcare providers to ensure ongoing surveillance and proactive adjustments to the treatment plan, if necessary.

3. Healthy Lifestyle Choices:
Embracing a healthy lifestyle contributes significantly to maintaining remission. This includes adopting a balanced diet, engaging in regular exercise, managing stress, and prioritizing sufficient sleep. Lifestyle choices play a synergistic role with medications in supporting overall well-being and preventing potential triggers for lupus flares.

1. Psychoeducational Support:
Psychoeducational support, encompassing educational resources and counseling services, helps individuals and their caregivers navigate the emotional challenges associated with lupus. Understanding the psychological impact of the disease, learning coping mechanisms, and accessing mental health resources contribute to emotional well-being.

2. Peer Assistance Systems:
Peer support networks play a pivotal role in coping with emotional challenges. Connecting with others who share similar experiences fosters a sense of community, understanding, and shared coping strategies. Peer support provides a valuable avenue for expressing emotions, seeking advice, and building resilience.

3. Individual and Family Counseling:
Individual and family counseling offer a structured space for addressing emotional challenges collaboratively. Individuals with lupus and their loved ones can benefit from sessions that provide tools for coping with stress, improving communication, and enhancing overall emotional resilience.

Navigating Relationships with Lupus

1. Open Communication with Loved Ones:
Open communication is key to navigating relationships when living with lupus. Individuals are encouraged to share their experiences, symptoms, and needs with their loved ones. Educating family and friends about lupus fosters empathy and creates a supportive environment.

2. Setting Boundaries:
Setting boundaries becomes crucial in managing relationships while coping with lupus. Clearly communicating personal limitations, expressing needs, and establishing boundaries help individuals strike a balance between social engagement and self-care. Loved ones play a vital role in respecting and supporting these boundaries.

3. Participation in Supportive Networks:
Participation in supportive networks extends beyond peer support to include family and friends. Involving loved ones in lupus education sessions, support groups, or family counseling sessions creates a shared understanding and strengthens the support system. The collective effort contributes to a more resilient and cohesive network.

Building a Support System

1. Identifying Key Supportive Individuals:
Building a support system involves identifying key individuals who play a supportive role. This may include family members, friends, healthcare providers, and members of the lupus community. Establishing clear lines of communication and recognizing the unique contributions of each support figure enhances the overall support network.

2. Educating Supportive Individuals:
Educating supportive individuals about lupus is essential for fostering understanding. Providing informational resources, attending medical appointments together, and involving loved ones in educational activities contribute to creating an informed and empathetic support system.

3. Utilizing Professional Support Services:
Professional support services, such as social workers or patient advocates, can be valuable additions to the support system. These professionals provide guidance on navigating healthcare systems, accessing resources, and addressing psychosocial aspects of living with lupus.

Future Perspectives on Coping with Flares and Remissions

1. Advancements in Personalized Medicine:
The future of lupus management involves advancements in personalized medicine. Tailored treatment plans, precision medicine approaches, and individualized interventions based on genetic and molecular profiles offer promising avenues for enhancing the effectiveness of treatment during flares and optimizing remission maintenance.

2. Innovations in Digital Health for Remote Monitoring:
Digital health innovations continue to transform lupus care. Remote monitoring through wearable devices, mobile apps, and telehealth platforms enables individuals and healthcare providers to closely track disease activity, medication adherence, and overall well-being. These innovations enhance real-time communication and proactive management strategies.

3. Expansion of Telehealth Services in Mental Health Support:
Telehealth services, particularly in mental health support, are expected to expand. Virtual counseling sessions, online support groups, and digital mental health

platforms provide convenient and accessible avenues for individuals with lupus to prioritize their emotional well-being. The integration of telehealth services ensures that mental health support remains a central component of lupus care, fostering resilience and coping strategies.

4. AI-driven Personalized Coping Plans:
Artificial Intelligence (AI) applications are poised to contribute to personalized coping plans. AI algorithms can analyze vast datasets, including individual health records, lifestyle factors, and psychological profiles. This analysis can result in the creation of personalized coping strategies that evolve based on real-time data, supporting individuals in managing flares and navigating remissions.

5. Community-Based Interventions:
Community-based interventions continue to be integral in future lupus care. Initiatives that focus on building strong community ties, fostering peer support, and promoting shared coping strategies become increasingly valuable. These interventions extend beyond traditional healthcare settings, emphasizing the role of community in holistic well-being.

6. Incorporation of Wearable Technology for Symptom Tracking:

Wearable technology evolves to play a more active role in tracking lupus symptoms. Advanced wearables may provide continuous monitoring of physiological markers, enabling individuals to detect subtle changes indicative of flares. The integration of these technologies empowers individuals to take proactive measures in managing their health.

7. Culturally Tailored Support Resources:
Future perspectives involve the development of culturally tailored support resources. Recognizing the diverse backgrounds and cultural influences within the lupus community, resources will be crafted to resonate with various cultural norms, beliefs, and preferences. Culturally sensitive support ensures inclusivity and relevance in coping strategies.

8. Empowerment through Self-Management Apps:
Self-management apps become increasingly sophisticated, offering interactive features that empower individuals to actively participate in their care. These apps may include modules for symptom tracking, personalized coping exercises, and educational content. The emphasis on user empowerment through technology becomes a cornerstone in coping with flares and optimizing well-being.

Embracing Resilience in the Lupus Journey

Chapter 10 delves into the intricate process of coping with flares and navigating periods of remission in the context of lupus. From identifying triggers and developing personalized response plans to engaging in supportive relationships and embracing innovative technologies, individuals with lupus are equipped with a comprehensive guide to managing the dynamic nature of the disease.

As we look toward the future, the landscape of coping with flares and remissions in lupus care continues to evolve. Advances in personalized medicine, digital health, and community-based interventions promise a more tailored and inclusive approach. The integration of technology, coupled with a holistic understanding of individual needs and cultural considerations, ensures that coping strategies remain dynamic, relevant, and empowering.

In the ongoing journey of living with lupus, individuals, caregivers, and healthcare providers collaborate to foster resilience, promote well-being, and navigate the complexities of the disease. By embracing the evolving perspectives outlined in this chapter, individuals with lupus can approach flares and remissions with confidence, informed decision-making, and a sense of empowerment, ultimately contributing to a higher quality of life on their lupus journey.

CHAPTER TEN

Coping with Lupus: Useful Advice

This chapter examines useful advice for people coping with the day-to-day difficulties of having lupus. This chapter offers insights that help people live fulfilling lives while managing the complexities of lupus, from creating a strong support network to overcoming emotional obstacles and managing relationships skillfully.

Establishing a Network of Support

1. Finding Crucial Support People:
Finding important people who fulfill supportive roles is the first step in creating a strong support network. Members of the lupus community, friends, family, and medical professionals can create a network of support.

Acknowledging the distinct contributions of every individual amplifies the overall robustness of the support structure.

2. Honest Communication
Building a support system requires effective communication at its core. People who have lupus should be honest about their needs, educate others about it, and let them know how others can be of real assistance. Transparent communication improves comprehension and fortifies ties within the support system.

3. Educating People Who Are Supportive:
It's crucial to inform people in the support system about lupus. Providing resources for information, going to doctor's appointments with loved ones, and including them in educational activities are all ways to build a knowledgeable and compassionate support network. Support people with lupus can take an active role in the disease by being educated.

Handling Emotional Difficulties

1. Obtaining Psychoeducational Materials:
Psychoeducational materials provide insightful advice on managing the emotional difficulties brought on by lupus. Information on comprehending emotions, fostering resilience, and creating coping mechanisms can be

found in books, articles, and internet resources. By using these tools, people can take charge of their emotional health.

2. Counseling, both individual and group:
Counseling, both individual and group, offers organized ways to deal with emotional problems. Expert counselors can help with stress management, coping strategy development, and navigating the psychological effects of having a chronic illness. An encouraging setting for exchanging experiences and picking up knowledge from others is provided by group counseling.

3. Techniques for Mindfulness:
Mental health benefits from mindfulness exercises like meditation and mindful breathing. These exercises improve resilience, lessen anxiety, and foster present-moment awareness. People can manage stress and foster emotional balance by incorporating mindfulness into their daily routines.

Managing Relationships

1. Clearly Delineating Boundaries:
When it comes to managing relationships while having lupus, setting clear boundaries is crucial. People can find

a balance between social interaction and self-care by expressing their needs, setting boundaries, and communicating their limitations. Maintaining and upholding these boundaries requires the support and respect of loved ones.

2. Teaching Our Loved Ones:
One proactive way to promote understanding is by educating family members and friends about lupus. Establishing a foundation of empathy and support involves providing information about the condition, its symptoms, and potential obstacles. When loved ones are informed about a person's experiences, they can become allies in their lupus journey.

3. Including Family Members in Medical Care:
Incorporating close ones into healthcare-related activities, like doctor visits or therapy conversations, fortifies the support network. By actively participating, family members can learn about lupus management, ask questions, and work with medical professionals to support the well-being of the individual.

Getting Along in Everyday Life

1. Modifying Office Spaces:
It is essential to modify work environments to meet health needs. People who have lupus should be upfront with employers regarding any modifications that are

required, like remote work choices, ergonomic accommodations, or flexible work schedules. These adjustments support a more favorable work-life balance.

2. Making Self-Care a Priority:
Making self-care a priority is essential to living a healthy, everyday life with lupus. A healthy diet, regular exercise, adequate sleep, and stress reduction all contribute to general wellbeing. Establishing a personalized self-care regimen guarantees that well-being is consistently prioritized in day-to-day activities.

3. Making Use of Assistive Devices:
The use of assistive technology can improve functionality and independence. Voice-activated technology, ergonomic tools, and mobility aids may be beneficial for people with lupus. By incorporating these tools into daily life, people can minimize the effects of their lupus symptoms while still managing tasks effectively.

Planning and Financial Aspects

1. Comprehending Benefits for Disability:
People who have lupus may investigate disability benefits in light of their medical condition. Comprehending the qualifying requirements, the application procedure, and the available resources guarantees financial security during times of limited

work ability. Seeking advice from a legal expert or disability advocate can help you through this process.

2. Organizing Your Money for Medical Expenses:
Examining insurance coverage, creating an out-of-pocket spending plan, and looking into financial aid options are all part of financial planning for medical costs. To reduce financial strain, people with lupus should plan ahead for medical expenses, such as prescription drugs, therapies, and routine check-ups.

3. Looking for Financial Advice:
Getting professional financial advice, such as from counselors or financial advisors, can offer valuable insights into managing finances while living with lupus. Financial stability is a result of developing a budget that takes individual needs into account, planning for future changes in income, and looking into available options.

Traveling while suffering from Lupus

1. Getting Ready and Making Plans:
When traveling, people with lupus need to plan ahead and prepare carefully. This entails setting up prescription drugs, health information, and required supplies. A more seamless travel experience can be achieved by

researching the destination's medical facilities, comprehending the coverage provided by travel insurance, and making backup plans.

2. Modifying Trip Schedules:
It is imperative to modify travel schedules to account for medical requirements. People who have lupus should prioritize rest, think about how climate change may affect their symptoms, and schedule their activities flexibly. Personalizing travel schedules minimizes physical strain while enabling a pleasurable experience.

3. Interaction with Travel Partners:
To ensure a supportive and enjoyable trip, it is essential to maintain open communication with fellow travelers. People who have lupus should talk to their travel companions about their needs, possible difficulties, and symptom management techniques. This kind of cooperation promotes mutual understanding and a cooperative way of traveling.

Effective Medication Management

1. Putting Medicines in Order:
A methodical approach to medication organization is necessary for effective medication management. Medication lists, pill organizers, and reminders all help with adherence. Patients with lupus ought to collaborate

with medical professionals to establish a medication regimen that complements their everyday activities.

2. Frequent Reviews of Medication:
Reviewing medications on a regular basis with medical professionals guarantees that the treatment plan is still appropriate and effective. During these reviews, people should actively communicate any changes in their symptoms, side effects, or medication-related concerns. Treatment plan modifications can be made cooperatively.

3. Emergency Medication Preparedness:
Preparedness for emergency situations involves having an accessible supply of essential medications. Creating an emergency medication kit with necessary prescriptions, contact information for healthcare providers, and clear instructions ensures that individuals can manage their health effectively during unforeseen circumstances.

Engaging in Hobbies and Leisure Activities

1. Identifying Enjoyable Hobbies:
Engaging in enjoyable hobbies contributes to overall well-being. Individuals with lupus should identify hobbies that align with their interests and are adaptable to their health needs. Whether it's reading, gardening,

or creative pursuits, hobbies provide avenues for relaxation and fulfillment.

2. Accessible Leisure Activities:
Accessible leisure activities cater to individual capabilities and health conditions. Individuals with lupus may explore activities such as gentle walks, seated exercises, or adaptive sports. Ensuring accessibility in leisure pursuits allows individuals to enjoy recreational activities while considering their unique physical comfort.

3. Participating in Community Events:
Involvement in community events fosters a sense of connection and engagement. Individuals with lupus can explore local events, support groups, or online communities related to their interests. Participating in these activities provides opportunities for social interaction, networking, and shared experiences.

Advocacy for Lupus Awareness

1. Personal Advocacy Efforts:
Personal advocacy involves sharing one's lupus journey to raise awareness. Individuals with lupus can participate in awareness campaigns, share their stories

through social media, or engage in community events. Personal advocacy contributes to dispelling myths, reducing stigma, and fostering understanding of lupus.

2. Participation in Support Groups:
Support groups offer a collective platform for advocacy efforts. Individuals with lupus can join or initiate support groups to share information, discuss challenges, and collectively advocate for better resources and understanding. Support groups become advocacy hubs within the lupus community.

3. Educating Healthcare Providers:
Educating healthcare providers about lupus is an impactful form of advocacy. Individuals can share informational materials, attend medical appointments with educational resources, and engage in open conversations about their experiences. This collaboration ensures that healthcare professionals are well-informed and supportive.

Balancing Parenthood and Lupus
1. Communication with Healthcare Providers:
Balancing parenthood and lupus requires open communication with healthcare providers. Individuals planning to start a family or those already parenting should discuss their intentions with their healthcare team. Healthcare providers can offer guidance on managing lupus during pregnancy and parenthood.

2. Creating Supportive Parenting Plans:
Creating supportive parenting plans involves collaborating with partners, family members, and healthcare providers. Individuals with lupus can develop strategies for managing fatigue, prioritizing self-care, and ensuring a supportive environment for both themselves and their children. Open communication within the family is essential.

3. Engaging in Parenting Communities:
Engaging in parenting communities, whether online or local, provides a supportive network. Connecting with other parents managing lupus allows for shared insights, advice, and mutual support. These communities become valuable resources for navigating the unique challenges of parenting with lupus.

Navigating Work and Lupus

1. Advocating for Workplace Accommodations:
Individuals with lupus are encouraged to advocate for workplace accommodations. This may include flexible work hours, ergonomic adjustments, or remote work options. Open communication with employers about health needs ensures a supportive work environment that accommodates the challenges of lupus.

2. Utilizing Employee Assistance Programs:

Employee Assistance Programs (EAPs) provide support for employees facing health challenges. Individuals with lupus can explore EAP resources, which may include counseling services, legal assistance, and wellness programs. Utilizing these programs contributes to overall well-being in the workplace.

3. Balancing Workload and Rest:
Balancing workload and rest is essential for individuals managing lupus in the workplace. Prioritizing tasks, taking scheduled breaks, and communicating with supervisors about health needs contribute to maintaining a sustainable work routine. Striking a balance ensures productivity while managing lupus symptoms.

Empowering the Lupus Community

1. Mentoring Newly Diagnosed Individuals:
Empowering the lupus community involves mentoring individuals who are newly diagnosed. Sharing experiences, providing guidance on coping strategies, and offering emotional support contribute to a sense of community resilience. Mentorship fosters a supportive environment for those navigating the initial stages of lupus.

2. Participating in Research Initiatives:
Active participation in lupus research initiatives
contributes to advancements in understanding and
treating the disease. Individuals with lupus can explore
opportunities to participate in clinical trials, share their
experiences through surveys, and contribute valuable
data to ongoing research efforts.

3. Collaborating with Advocacy Organizations:
Collaboration with lupus advocacy organizations
amplifies individual voices and efforts. Individuals can
join or support advocacy groups, participate in
awareness campaigns, and engage in initiatives that aim
to improve resources, policies, and public understanding
of lupus.

Future Perspectives on Living with Lupus

1. Advancements in Treatment Options:
The future holds promising advancements in treatment
options for lupus. Ongoing research explores novel
therapies, precision medicine approaches, and targeted
interventions. These advancements aim to improve
treatment effectiveness, minimize side effects, and

provide more tailored solutions for individuals with lupus.

2. Enhancements in Remote Healthcare Access:
Enhancements in remote healthcare access continue to evolve, offering individuals with lupus more convenient and accessible options. Telehealth services, virtual monitoring, and online support platforms contribute to improved healthcare management from the comfort of one's home.

3. Integration of AI in Personalized Care Plans:
The integration of Artificial Intelligence (AI) in healthcare holds promise for personalized care plans. AI applications may analyze individual health data, predict potential disease patterns, and offer tailored recommendations for managing lupus. This innovation aims to enhance individualized care and treatment outcomes.

4. Expansion of Peer Support Networks:
Peer support networks are expected to expand, providing more opportunities for individuals with lupus to connect, share experiences, and offer mutual support. Online platforms, virtual support groups, and innovative peer-led initiatives contribute to the growth of these valuable networks.

5. Inclusive Workplace Policies:

In the future, workplace policies are anticipated to become more inclusive and accommodating for individuals managing chronic health conditions, including lupus. Employers may adopt policies that prioritize flexibility, understanding, and proactive support for employees facing health challenges.

6. Holistic Approaches in Mainstream Medicine:
Holistic approaches, including integrative medicine and lifestyle interventions, are expected to gain more recognition in mainstream lupus care. Healthcare providers may increasingly incorporate complementary therapies, nutritional guidance, and mental health support into comprehensive lupus management plans.

Advocacy and Awareness: A Lifelong Commitment

1. Continuous Education and Awareness:
Lifelong advocacy involves a commitment to continuous education and awareness. Staying informed about the latest developments in lupus research, treatment options, and support resources allows individuals to

advocate more effectively. Engaging in ongoing learning contributes to empowered decision-making.

2. Utilizing Social Media for Advocacy:
Social media platforms offer powerful tools for advocacy. Individuals with lupus can utilize these platforms to share personal stories, disseminate accurate information, and connect with a broader audience. Leveraging social media fosters a virtual community that raises awareness and provides support.

3. Participating in Public Awareness Campaigns:
Actively participating in public awareness campaigns contributes to broader efforts in educating the general population about lupus. Joining initiatives such as Lupus Awareness Month, organizing local events, and collaborating with advocacy organizations amplify individual voices in the collective mission to increase lupus awareness.

Ongoing Personal Development

1. Embracing Lifelong Learning:
Lifelong learning remains a key aspect of personal development. Individuals with lupus can explore educational opportunities, whether formal or informal, to enhance their knowledge and skills. Pursuing interests and acquiring new insights contributes to personal growth and resilience.

2. Exploring Adaptive Hobbies:
As interests evolve, individuals with lupus can explore adaptive hobbies that align with their capabilities. Whether it's learning a new instrument, engaging in artistic pursuits, or discovering technology-driven hobbies, adaptive activities provide avenues for creativity and enjoyment.

3. Mental and Emotional Wellness Practices:
Prioritizing mental and emotional wellness practices is an ongoing commitment. Regular engagement in mindfulness activities, seeking counseling when needed, and actively participating in emotional well-being strategies contribute to a resilient mindset. Fostering mental and emotional wellness remains a lifelong journey.

Nurturing Supportive Relationships

1. Building Deeper Connections:
Lifelong relationships evolve as individuals and circumstances change. Nurturing supportive relationships involves building deeper connections with loved ones, friends, and members of the lupus community. Open communication, empathy, and mutual understanding strengthen the fabric of these relationships.

2. Adapting to Life Changes:
Adapting to life changes is a continuous process. As
individuals with lupus navigate various stages in life,
including parenthood, career transitions, or retirement,
adapting to these changes requires flexibility and
resilience. The support system plays a crucial role in
facilitating these adjustments.

3. Mutual Growth in Relationships:
Relationships have the potential for mutual growth as
individuals learn and evolve together. Embracing shared
experiences, learning from challenges, and celebrating
achievements contribute to the overall growth of
relationships. The journey of living with lupus becomes a
shared narrative within supportive networks.

Exploring New Frontiers in Treatment

1. Participation in Clinical Trials:
Lifelong engagement with treatment options may
involve exploring participation in clinical trials.
Individuals with lupus can contribute to advancing
medical knowledge and gaining access to cutting-edge
treatments by participating in well-designed clinical
trials. Consultation with healthcare providers is crucial in
making informed decisions.

2. Advocating for Research Funding:
Advocacy efforts extend to advocating for increased research funding for lupus. Individuals can participate in initiatives that call for more funding, engage with policymakers, and support organizations working toward advancing lupus research. Increased research funding holds the potential for transformative breakthroughs.

3. Staying Informed about Treatment Advances:
Staying informed about treatment advances is integral to proactive healthcare management. Regular communication with healthcare providers, attending medical conferences, and accessing reputable sources of information ensure that individuals are aware of emerging treatment options and can make informed decisions about their care.

Holistic Well-being Across the Lifespan

1. Tailoring Lifestyle Adjustments:
Lifestyle adjustments remain dynamic and adaptable throughout the lifespan. As individuals age, the need for tailored lifestyle adjustments may evolve. Collaborating with healthcare providers to reassess and tailor strategies ensures that lifestyle adjustments effectively address changing needs.

2. Promoting Healthy Aging:

Promoting healthy aging involves a holistic approach to well-being. Maintaining a balanced diet, engaging in regular exercise appropriate for one's health condition, and prioritizing mental and emotional wellness contribute to healthy aging. Collaborative discussions with healthcare providers support individuals in embracing the aging process with resilience.

3. Cultivating a Positive Outlook:
Cultivating a positive outlook is a lifelong mindset. Despite the challenges of living with lupus, fostering optimism, gratitude, and a sense of purpose contributes to overall well-being. Actively seeking positive experiences, building resilience, and embracing life with a positive mindset enhance the quality of life.

Chapter 11 has provided practical tips for individuals living with lupus, emphasizing the importance of building a robust support system, managing emotional challenges, navigating relationships, and thriving in various aspects of daily life. As we look towards the future, the ongoing commitment to advocacy, continuous personal development, nurturing supportive relationships, exploring new frontiers in treatment, and promoting holistic well-being across the lifespan define a lifelong journey of resilience and growth.

Living with lupus involves adapting, learning, and evolving, but it also encompasses the strength to face challenges head-on and the capacity to lead a fulfilling life. The journey is marked by milestones, setbacks, and continuous self-discovery. Through proactive engagement with various aspects of life, individuals with lupus can not only manage the complexities of the condition but also embrace a life rich in meaning, connection, and well-being.

Chapter 11: Women and Lupus

Lupus, a complex autoimmune disease, affects individuals across many demographics, but its impact on women introduces special considerations that entangle with reproductive and hormonal elements of life. In this chapter, we explore into the obstacles and hardships women encounter, addressing themes ranging from lupus and pregnancy to menopause and hormonal shifts.

Lupus and Pregnancy

Navigating the Journey

Women with lupus typically embark on a special journey when considering pregnancy. The connection between the autoimmune illness and pregnancy provides both obstacles and opportunity. Consulting with a rheumatologist and an obstetrician who specialize in high-risk pregnancies becomes vital for a well-informed and supportive decision-making process.

Risks and Management

Pregnancy in the presence of lupus requires cautious monitoring due to potential difficulties. Increased risks of preterm birth, hypertension, and fetal development limitation demand attentive medical supervision. Balancing drugs to control lupus symptoms while protecting the safety of the unborn child offers a sensitive challenge, stressing the necessity for a coordinated healthcare strategy.

Postpartum Considerations

The postpartum phase offers its own set of considerations. Understanding the potential impact of hormonal variations on lupus activity is critical. Postpartum flares are not commonplace, and women need support in maintaining their health while caring for a newborn.

Menopause and Hormonal Changes

Shifting Dynamics

As women with lupus migrate into menopause, the hormonal landscape undergoes dramatic alterations.

Estrogen, which can have immunomodulatory effects, undergoes a reduction. This transition may alter lupus symptoms, with some women noting variations in disease activity.

Managing Symptoms

Navigating menopause with lupus demands personalized tactics. Addressing symptoms such as joint pain, exhaustion, and mood fluctuations becomes crucial. Hormone replacement treatment (HRT), typically utilized to manage menopausal symptoms, should be approached cautiously and under the advice of healthcare specialists due to its potential impact on lupus.

Emotional Well-being

Menopause might also cause emotional issues. Coping with changes in self-image, resolving concerns about fertility, and transitioning to a different period of life can be emotionally difficult. Support groups and mental health resources play a significant role in helping women handle these issues.

Women and Lupus

Fertility and Family Planning

For women with lupus contemplating family planning, reproductive considerations add another degree of complexity. Some drugs used to control lupus symptoms may influence fertility, necessitating deliberate talks with healthcare practitioners. Fertility specialists can offer insights into assisted reproductive technologies as needed, ensuring educated decisions fit with both health and family goals.

Support Networks

Building a robust support system is crucial for women managing lupus-related issues. Connecting with other women who share similar experiences gives a sense of camaraderie. Support groups, both online and in-person, offer platforms for exchanging thoughts, coping skills, and emotional support. Establishing a network of understanding friends and family members also leads to a more resilient trip.

Getting Around Intimate Relationships

Lupus can impair personal relationships, affecting both physical and emotional elements. Open conversation with partners regarding the impact of lupus on intimacy is vital. Education and counseling can assist couples in navigating these transitions, establishing a supportive and understanding environment.

Menopause and Beyond: Adapting to Change

Bone Health

Postmenopausal women with lupus confront additional considerations linked to bone health. Osteoporosis, commonly related with lupus and aggravated by hormonal changes during menopause, demands treatment. Adequate calcium consumption, vitamin D supplementation, and weight-bearing workouts contribute to maintaining bone density.

Cardiovascular Health

As women mature, cardiovascular health becomes a focal issue. Lupus itself can increase the risk of cardiovascular complications, and menopause adds additional layer to this concern. Lifestyle adjustments, such as a heart-healthy diet and regular exercise, are key components of reducing cardiovascular risk in women with lupus.

Hormone Replacement Therapy (HRT) Revisited

The decision to undertake hormone replacement treatment (HRT) during menopause should be reviewed post-diagnosis of lupus. While HRT can reduce menopausal symptoms, its impact on lupus activity requires cautious assessment. Consultation with both rheumatologists and gynecologists aids in building a specific approach to managing menopausal symptoms without compromising lupus care.

Empowering Women with Knowledge

Empowering women with lupus entails providing comprehensive education and resources. This chapter strives to empower women with the knowledge needed to make informed decisions at various phases of life. By embracing a holistic perspective that includes medical, emotional, and social components, women can manage the complexity of life with lupus with strength and confidence.

In conclusion, this chapter underlines the necessity of acknowledging the particular obstacles women with lupus confront throughout their life. By developing awareness, providing support, and delivering individualized medical counsel, we seek to encourage women to lead productive lives despite the challenges imposed by lupus. As we continue to explore the subtleties of lupus and its confluence with women's health, the shared knowledge becomes a beacon, directing women on a path towards optimal well-being.

CHAPTER TWELVE

Pediatric Lupus

Lupus, typically seen as an adult-onset autoimmune illness, also affects a subgroup of the population that is often overlooked—children and adolescents. This chapter addresses the special issues, problems, and methods related with pediatric lupus, putting emphasis on the importance of family support and available resources.

Unique Considerations for Children and Adolescents

Early-Onset Lupus

Pediatric lupus presents special issues due to its early onset. Children may struggle to describe their symptoms, necessitating alert parents and healthcare practitioners attuned to small changes. The signs of lupus in children can differ from those in adults, demanding specific care and diagnostic techniques.

Impact on Growth and Development

Lupus can impact a child's growth and development. Chronic inflammation, drugs, and the emotional toll of living with a chronic illness can contribute to delays in physical and emotional growth. Multidisciplinary care combining rheumatologists, pediatricians, and developmental specialists is vital for tackling these complicated concerns.

Educational Implications

Managing lupus while pursuing education needs teamwork between families, schools, and healthcare providers. Fatigue, cognitive issues, and the necessity for frequent medical appointments can influence a child's academic performance. Establishing a complete plan that incorporates school accommodations and support services offers an ideal learning environment.

Family Support and Resources

The Role of Parents and Caregivers

Parents of children with lupus play a vital role in managing the condition. They become activists, caregivers, and emotional support networks. Balancing the challenges of caring for a kid with lupus while meeting the needs of the entire family requires perseverance and adaptability.

Supportive Networks for Families

Connecting with other families facing similar struggles gives a sense of community and shared understanding. Support groups targeted to pediatric lupus offer significant insights, resources, and emotional support. Online forums and local meet-ups can foster these interactions, lowering feelings of loneliness for both children and their families.

Pediatric Lupus Organizations

Several organizations focus exclusively on pediatric lupus, offering a plethora of resources and support. These organizations play a significant role in advocacy, research financing, and providing instructional resources. By actively engaging with these entities, families can stay informed about the latest breakthroughs in pediatric lupus care.

Collaborative Care and Medical Management

Pediatric Rheumatologists and Multidisciplinary Teams

Pediatric lupus management requires a particular strategy, often led by pediatric rheumatologists. These experts collaborate with a multidisciplinary team, including pediatric nephrologists, dermatologists, and other specialists as needed. This comprehensive approach guarantees that the particular characteristics of pediatric lupus, such as renal involvement or cutaneous symptoms, are adequately handled.

Medications and Adverse Effects

Managing lupus in children includes carefully balancing the benefits of drugs with potential negative effects. Corticosteroids, immunosuppressants, and antimalarials are among the often recommended drugs. Pediatric rheumatologists regularly monitor medication effects and adapt treatment plans to prevent adverse responses, understanding the significance of promoting the child's general well-being.

Transitioning to Adult Care

As adolescents with lupus graduate to adulthood, navigating the transfer from pediatric to adult care is a key milestone. This approach entails training individuals for more responsibility in managing their health while enabling a smooth transfer of medical information and communication between pediatric and adult healthcare providers.

Family Dynamics and Emotional Well-being

Sibling Relationships

The impact of pediatric lupus extends beyond the afflicted child to siblings. Siblings may experience a range of emotions, from concern for their brother or sister to feelings of neglect due to greater focus on the child with lupus. Open communication within the family encourages understanding and support among siblings.

Emotional Resilience

Pediatric lupus can be emotionally hard for both children and their families. Coping with the uncertainties of a chronic illness, potential lifestyle limits, and the emotional toll of medical treatments demands emotional resilience. Psychosocial support, including counseling and mental health resources, is vital to the well-being of the entire family.

Balancing Normalcy and Adaptation

Fostering a feeling of normalcy within the family dynamic is vital. While adapting to the specific challenges of pediatric lupus, families seek to preserve routines, acknowledge achievements, and create pleasant experiences. Encouraging children with lupus to engage in age-appropriate activities increases sociability and a sense of belonging.

Advocacy for Pediatric Lupus

Raising Awareness

Advocacy plays a critical role in improving outcomes for children with lupus. Raising awareness about pediatric lupus among the general public, healthcare practitioners, and lawmakers is crucial for greater research funding, access to specialist care, and the development of tailored medicines.

Family Advocacy

Parents and caregivers become champions not only for their kid but also for the greater pediatric lupus community. Participating in advocacy initiatives, supporting research efforts, and sharing personal stories contribute to a collective voice that drives good change.

Conclusion

In this chapter, we have looked into the special concerns regarding pediatric lupus, emphasizing the need of family support, collaborative medical care, and activism. Recognizing the obstacles faced by children and adolescents with lupus and their families is a vital step toward promoting understanding and improving outcomes.

By addressing the numerous facets of juvenile lupus, from educational implications to emotional well-being, this chapter strives to provide a comprehensive resource for families navigating this complicated path. The fortitude displayed by children and their families in the face of lupus serves as a monument to the strength of the human spirit and the power of support networks.

As we continue to increase our understanding of pediatric lupus and enhance the tools available, the ultimate goal is to empower families to handle the obstacles with knowledge, resilience, and a feeling of community. In doing so, we contribute to a brighter future for children and adolescents living with lupus, ensuring that they can lead full lives despite the complications of their health journey.

CHAPTER THIRTEEN

Advocacy and Awareness

Advocacy and awareness are crucial in the arena of lupus, where understanding, support, and action can profoundly improve the lives of persons impacted by this complex autoimmune disease. This chapter addresses the role of advocacy, both at the individual and community levels, and stresses the significance of raising awareness to encourage positive change.

Being a Proponent for Your own self and Others

Self-Advocacy in Healthcare

Empowering persons with lupus to be advocates for their own health is a vital element of controlling the condition. This requires active engagement in medical decisions, clear communication with healthcare providers, and being educated about treatment options. Building a collaborative connection with medical providers ensures tailored care that matches with individual requirements and preferences.

Seeking Second Opinions

Navigating the difficulties of lupus typically entails getting second views. As the condition manifests differently in each individual, exploring multiple perspectives from medical specialists might offer significant insights and alternate ways to treatment. Encouraging a proactive attitude to healthcare decisions adds to informed choices and a sense of control over one's health.

Accessing Support Services

Being an advocate for oneself also goes to receiving support resources. From patient assistance programs that provide financial support for drugs to community services offering emotional and practical assistance, patients with lupus benefit from recognizing and utilizing the available support networks.

Raising Lupus Awareness in the Community

The Power of Personal Stories

Sharing personal tales is an effective strategy for spreading lupus awareness. Individuals affected by lupus, together with their family and caregivers, can contribute to destigmatizing the disease by sharing their stories. These stories humanize lupus, creating empathy and understanding within the broader community.

Social Media and Online Platforms

In the digital age, social media and online platforms play a key role in promoting awareness. Advocacy groups, individuals, and healthcare organizations employ these platforms to exchange information, dispel myths, and develop supportive networks. The reach of online platforms extends globally, uniting individuals and generating a sense of unity.

Organizing Local Events

Community-based events provide practical chances to increase awareness. Local walks, fundraisers, and educational seminars not only involve the community but also give venues for those with lupus to share their stories. Collaborating with local companies, schools, and healthcare professionals multiplies the effect of these activities.

Being a Voice for Change

Advocacy Initiatives

Engaging in advocacy campaigns is vital for affecting systemic change. Individuals and organizations engaged to lupus advocacy fight towards more research funding, improved access to healthcare, and policy changes that benefit the lupus community. Participation in advocacy days, contacting political officials, and supporting legislative efforts are effective ways to be a voice for change.

Collaborating with Healthcare Professionals

Building ties with healthcare professionals boosts the effectiveness of lupus advocacy. Collaborative efforts between patients, advocacy organizations, and medical specialists contribute to a unified voice that can impact healthcare legislation, research goals, and access to novel therapies.

International Collaboration

Lupus knows no borders, and international collaboration is crucial for addressing the global effect of the disease. Participating in international conferences, sponsoring global research projects, and promoting cross-cultural encounters contribute to a collective effort to enhance lupus awareness and research.

Promoting Diversity and Inclusivity in Lupus Advocacy

Addressing Disparities in Healthcare

Lupus disproportionately affects specific populations, and advocacy initiatives must address healthcare disparities. Raising awareness about the impact of lupus on varied groups, advocating for culturally competent healthcare, and addressing social determinants of health contribute to a more inclusive and equitable approach to lupus advocacy.

Supporting Underrepresented Groups

Empowering underrepresented groups within the lupus community is vital to effective advocacy. Tailoring awareness efforts, support services, and research activities to reflect the unique needs of varied groups ensures that no one is left behind in the pursuit of enhanced lupus care and understanding.

Cultural Competence in Advocacy

Cultural competence in lupus advocacy requires recognizing and respecting diverse views, traditions, and experiences. Cultivating an inclusive atmosphere where persons from various backgrounds feel heard and understood boosts the lupus advocacy network and broadens its effect.

Advocacy Challenges and Strategies

Overcoming Stigma

Stigma surrounding lupus can hamper advocacy efforts. Misconceptions about the condition may lead to discrimination and lack of understanding. Advocacy activities must target and confront these stigmas, offering correct information and developing understanding.

Bridging Gaps in Research Funding

Research funding is vital for expanding lupus knowledge and treatment options. Advocates work towards reducing gaps in research funding by interacting with lawmakers, raising public awareness about the need for more investment, and supporting initiatives that prioritize lupus research.

Navigating Legislative Processes

Navigating legislative processes demands a smart strategy. Advocates interact with policymakers, provide evidence-based information, and mobilize grassroots support to influence legislative decisions that impact the lupus community. Understanding the legislative landscape and creating relationships with decision-makers are crucial components of successful advocacy.

Future Directions in Lupus Advocacy

Technological Advances

Advances in technology give new chances for lupus advocacy. Virtual platforms, mobile applications, and telehealth services offer creative methods to connect, educate, and organize the lupus community. Embracing these technology tools boosts the reach and impact of lobbying activities.

Integrating Mental Health Advocacy

Addressing mental health in lupus advocacy is getting recognition. The emotional toll of living with a chronic condition is considerable, and adding mental health advocacy with lupus programs promotes a comprehensive approach to well-being. Destigmatizing mental health discussions within the lupus community leads to a supportive atmosphere.

Long-Term Sustainability

Ensuring the long-term viability of lupus advocacy demands strategic planning and community engagement. Building networks of dedicated advocates, creating leadership within the lupus community, and developing sustainable funding strategies contribute to a robust and durable advocacy movement.

Conclusion

Advocacy and awareness are catalysts for good change in the landscape of lupus. From self-advocacy in healthcare to raising community awareness, individuals and groups play crucial roles in crafting a future where lupus is better understood, well-supported, and effectively managed.

This chapter serves as a call to action, encouraging those afflicted by lupus, healthcare professionals, and the larger community to actively engage in advocacy initiatives. By elevating voices, refuting myths, and fostering collaborative projects, we can jointly contribute to a future where lupus is met with understanding, compassion, and comprehensive assistance. Through ongoing advocacy, we pave the path for improvements in research, increased healthcare access, and eventually, a brighter future for those living with lupus.

CHAPTER FOURTEEN

Future Perspectives and Resources

As we stand at the confluence of the present and the future in lupus research and care, this chapter digs into the dynamic landscape of improvements, continuous support services, and the hope of breakthroughs. Looking ahead, we evaluate the current state of lupus research, the resources available for continued support, and the potential future approaches that may change the understanding and therapy of this complicated autoimmune illness.

Current Lupus Research and Breakthroughs

Immunological Insights

Advancements in immunological research are providing deeper insights into the underlying mechanisms of lupus. Understanding the complicated relationships between the immune system components offers light on potential targets for therapeutic therapies. From the significance of individual cells to the signaling pathways involved in lupus pathogenesis, current study leads to a more comprehensive grasp of the illness.

Precision Medicine Approaches

The era of precision medicine promises hope for tailored lupus care. Genetic and molecular profiling allow for individualized treatment regimens, reflecting the unique aspects of each patient's condition. Identifying biomarkers related with lupus activity offers more accurate diagnosis and surveillance, paving the door for tailored therapy strategies.

Targeted Therapies in Development

The pharmaceutical landscape for lupus is shifting with the emergence of tailored treatments. Monoclonal antibodies and small chemical inhibitors targeted to selectively alter immune responses are undergoing clinical testing. These innovative treatments attempt to improve efficacy while limiting adverse effects, offering new pathways for managing lupus symptoms.

Advancements in Treatment Delivery

In addition to innovative therapeutic drugs, innovations in treatment delivery systems are being studied. Subcutaneous and oral formulations, as opposed to typical intravenous administration, promote convenience and accessibility for patients. These improvements aim to optimize treatment adherence and improve the overall patient experience.

Patient-Reported Outcomes in Research

Patient-reported outcomes (PROs) are gaining popularity in lupus research. Capturing the patient's perspective on disease impact, symptomatology, and treatment effects provides significant data for clinical studies and healthcare decision-making. Incorporating PROs ensures a full understanding of the patient experience, supporting patient-centered treatment.

Ongoing Support Resources

Patient Education and Empowerment

Patient education is a cornerstone of lupus management. Resources that empower individuals with information about their disease, treatment alternatives, and lifestyle factors assist to informed decision-making. Educational tools, online courses, and workshops play significant roles in strengthening the health literacy of the lupus community.

Support Groups and Networks

Support groups continue to be vital to the lupus community, providing emotional support, shared experiences, and practical advice. Both in-person and online support networks establish areas where persons with lupus, their families, and caregivers may interact, share insights, and manage the obstacles of living with the disease.

Nonprofit Organizations

Nonprofit groups committed to lupus advocacy and support are crucial in offering resources and encouraging positive change. These organizations offer a range of services, including financial aid programs, educational resources, and activities focused on promoting awareness. Collaborating with and supporting these organizations enhances the collective effect of the lupus community.

Telehealth and Remote Care

Advancements in telehealth and remote care boost accessibility to healthcare services for patients with lupus. Virtual consultations, remote monitoring, and digital health platforms provide continued care and support, particularly for persons suffering geographical or mobility constraints.

Educational Symposia and Conferences

Symposia and conferences focused on lupus provide forums for knowledge sharing, collaboration, and professional growth. These events bring together researchers, healthcare professionals, and persons impacted by lupus, providing a collaborative environment that accelerates progress in research and care.

Anticipated Future Perspectives

Emerging Technologies in Diagnosis

The future promises the possibility of more efficient and accurate diagnostic instruments. Advances in imaging technology, biomarker identification, and artificial intelligence applications may change the early detection of lupus, enabling prompt therapies and improved results.

Personalized Treatment Plans

Continued breakthroughs in precision medicine may lead to additional tailored treatment strategies. Tailoring approaches based on an individual's genetic profile, immune system features, and sensitivity to certain therapies could improve lupus care, enhancing outcomes and minimizing adverse effects.

Gene Editing and Therapeutic Advancements

Gene editing tools, such as CRISPR-Cas9, present new avenues for therapeutic breakthroughs. Precision editing of genes related with lupus susceptibility or disease development holds the potential to address root causes, giving transformational approaches to treatment.

Regenerative Medicine Approaches

Exploration of regenerative medicine in lupus focuses on repairing or replacing damaged tissues. Stem cell therapies and tissue engineering hold promise for restoring function in organs impaired by lupus, potentially delivering long-term benefits beyond symptom control.

Integrative Healthcare Models

The future may witness an increased fusion of conventional and unconventional healthcare practices. Integrative models that combine conventional medical treatments with alternative therapies, such as acupuncture or nutritional therapy, try to accommodate the different requirements of individuals with lupus.

Conclusion

As we peek into the future of lupus research and care, the picture appears both hopeful and dynamic. Ongoing research activities, advancements in treatment methods, and an ever-expanding array of support resources collectively contribute to a positive outlook for persons affected with lupus.

This chapter stresses the necessity of being informed, engaged, and connected within the lupus community. Whether through involvement in clinical trials, accessing novel treatment options, or contributing to advocacy activities, individuals with lupus play active roles in defining the future of lupus care.

The journey ahead entails a collective effort that encompasses scholars, healthcare professionals, advocacy organizations, and, most importantly, those living with lupus. By promoting a culture of resilience, empowerment, and constant learning, we collectively pave the way for a future where lupus is not only better understood and managed but also where persons affected by lupus lead lives filled with hope, support, and optimal well-being.

CHAPTER FIFTHEEN

Customized Approaches to Lupus

Treatment

Due to its high degree of variability and complexity, lupus requires individualized treatment plans that take into consideration patient differences in symptoms, disease presentations, and general health. This chapter examines various treatment options according to particular lupus conditions, highlighting recommended medications and treatments that medical practitioners may take into account when creating individualized management plans.

Overarching Concepts of Lupus Management

Immunosuppressive Drugs

Immunosuppressive drugs are the mainstay of care for lupus. They function by regulating the immune system's hyperactivity, which lowers the risk of organ damage and helps to control inflammation. Typical immunosuppressants consist of:

- Mycophenolate Mofetil (CellCept): Often used in lupus nephritis, this medication is effective in suppressing immune cell activity.

- Azathioprine (Imuran): Used to treat a variety of lupus symptoms, this medication helps control inflammation.

- Cyclophosphamide, also known as Cytoxan: Used in cases of severe lupus, particularly lupus nephritis.

Corticosteroids

Strong anti-inflammatory medications called corticosteroids, like prednisone, are used to treat lupus flare-ups. Even though it works well, prolonged use can have negative effects, which is why it's crucial to reduce dosage whenever feasible.

Antimalarial Medication

Plaquenil, also known as hydroxychloroquine, is frequently prescribed to treat lupus symptoms. It is especially useful for skin and joint symptoms because of its anti-inflammatory qualities.

NSAIDs, or nonsteroidal anti-inflammatory drugs,

NSAIDs like ibuprofen may be prescribed to treat mild joint and muscle pain in order to reduce symptoms.

Customized Strategies Depending on Lupus Symptoms

lupus arthritis

Immunosuppressive drugs are often used in combination to treat lupus nephritis, a severe kidney symptom. These could be rituximab, cyclophosphamide, or mycophenolate mofetil. Monitoring kidney function closely is essential for the treatment of lupus nephritis.

Lupus Cutaneous

Treatment options for cutaneous lupus, a type of lupus that manifests as skin symptoms, include topical corticosteroids, antimalarial medications, and sun protection techniques. Systemic drugs like dapsone or methotrexate may be taken into consideration in situations where there is more severe skin involvement.

The Joint Pain and Arthritis

Nonsteroidal anti-inflammatory drugs (NSAIDs) are frequently used for symptomatic relief of arthritis and joint pain in lupus patients. For more thorough treatment, disease-modifying antirheumatic medications (DMARDs) like methotrexate or hydroxychloroquine may be added.

Heart-related Involvement

Reducing cardiovascular risks in lupus patients requires changing lifestyle habits and taking medicine to control high blood pressure and cholesterol. Because of its antiplatelet properties, aspirin may be advised, and in some circumstances, anticoagulants may be taken into consideration.

Lupus neuropsychiatric

Handling central nervous system involvement in neuropsychiatric lupus necessitates a multidisciplinary approach. The treatment plan may include immunosuppressants, corticosteroids, and drugs that target particular symptoms (such as antiepileptic drugs for seizures).

Chest Involvement

Corticosteroids and immunosuppressive medications may be prescribed for lung conditions associated with lupus, such as pleuritis or pulmonary hypertension. Medication aimed at pulmonary hypertension or oxygen therapy might also be taken into consideration.

Recommended Medications and Treatments for Symptomatic Relief

Handling Exhaustion

One of the common challenges of lupus is chronic fatigue. Pacing activities, implementing regular rest periods, and making sure you get enough sleep are some strategies. Although there isn't a specific medication for fatigue, treating underlying lupus activity and related disorders may help reduce fatigue.

Handling Photosensitivity

Wearing protective clothing, avoiding the hottest parts of the day, and applying sunscreen with a high SPF can all help manage photosensitivity, a common problem in lupus. In addition to alleviating skin symptoms, antimalarial medications such as hydroxychloroquine also aid in photoprotection.

Dealing with Hair Loss

The unsettling symptom of lupus, hair loss, may get better with antimalarial medications. Topical minoxidil is a possibility, and it's best to speak with a dermatologist for specific advice.

Handling Joint Pain

NSAIDs may provide momentary relief from joint pain associated with lupus. Individualized low-impact exercises and physical therapy can support the preservation of joint function. Disease-modifying antirheumatic medications (DMARDs) may be taken into consideration for chronic joint problems.

Comprehensive Methods for Lupus Treatment

• Nutritional Aspects

Although a specific diet for lupus does not exist, adhering to an anti-inflammatory, well-balanced diet may benefit general health. Fish oil contains omega-3 fatty acids, which may have anti-inflammatory properties. A few lupus sufferers find relief from flare-ups by avoiding specific foods.

• Health and Physical Exercise

Personalized exercise regimens are essential for managing lupus. Walking, yoga, and other low-impact exercises can help increase joint flexibility and general health. Consistently engaging in mild physical activity can help preserve bodily functions.

Techniques for Stress Management

Flares of lupus may be exacerbated by prolonged stress. Controlling symptoms may be aided by stress management strategies like mindfulness, meditation, or relaxation training. Consulting with mental health specialists can also be helpful.

Working Together to Make Decisions with Healthcare Providers

People with lupus and their healthcare providers must work together to choose the right medications and treatments. Effective lupus care necessitates regular communication, symptom monitoring, and plan modifications based on patient responses.

In summary

The significance of customizing lupus treatment according to the various disease manifestations is emphasized in this chapter. Understanding that every person with lupus is different, medical professionals collaborate with patients to create individualized treatment programs. Improving quality of life, preventing organ damage, and optimizing symptom control are the objectives, which may involve immunosuppressive drugs and lifestyle changes.

People who have lupus are advised to actively participate in conversations with their medical professionals, offering personal perspectives on their symptoms and encounters. People with lupus become partners in their care by encouraging open communication and actively taking part in treatment decisions. This helps to create a more thorough and individualized approach to managing this complex autoimmune condition.

Made in the USA
Las Vegas, NV
13 May 2024

89854006R00095